Biomedical Signal and Image Processing

Edited by Yongxia Zhou

Published in London, United Kingdom

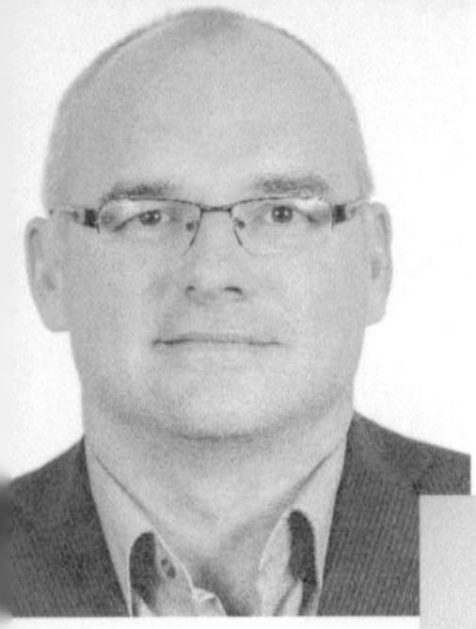
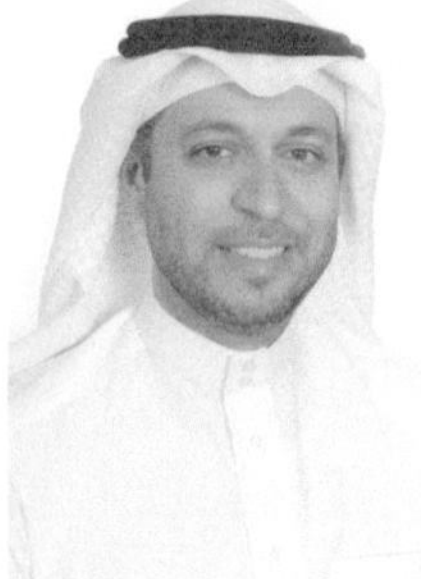
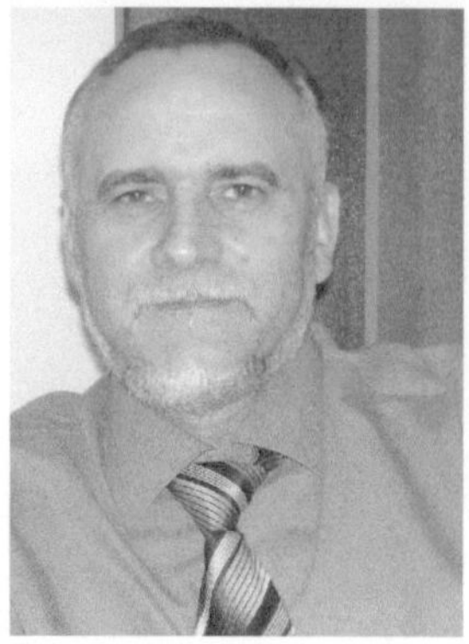
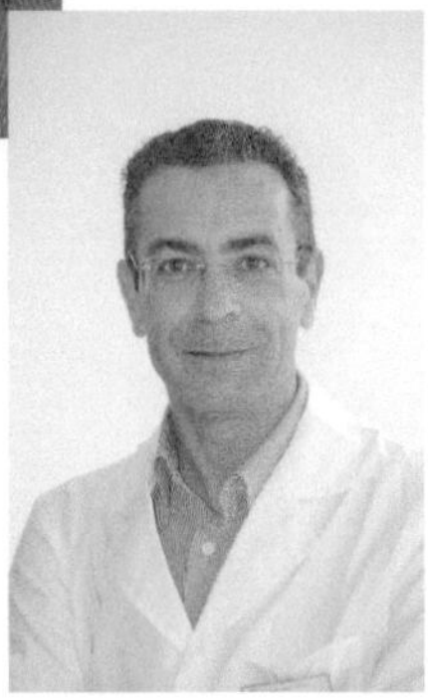
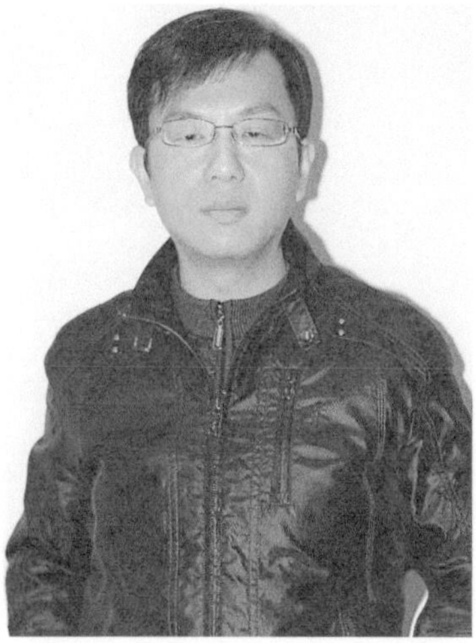
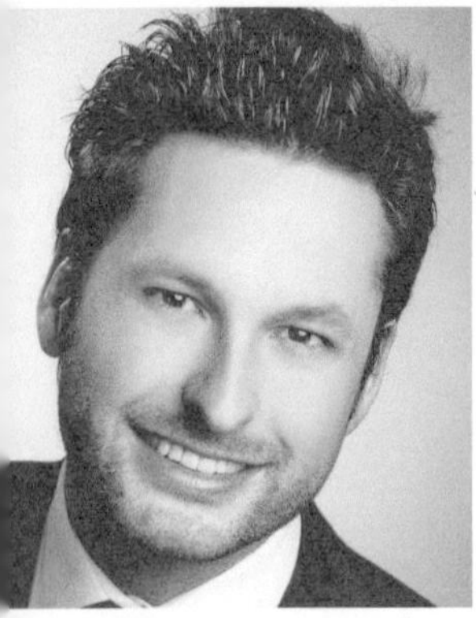
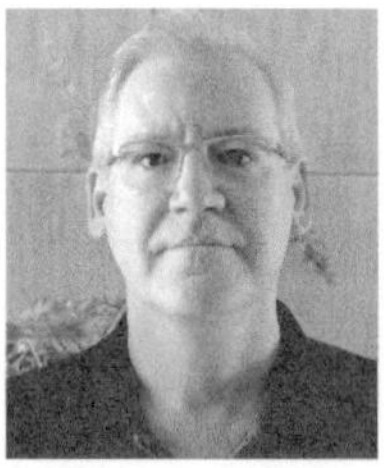

IntechOpen

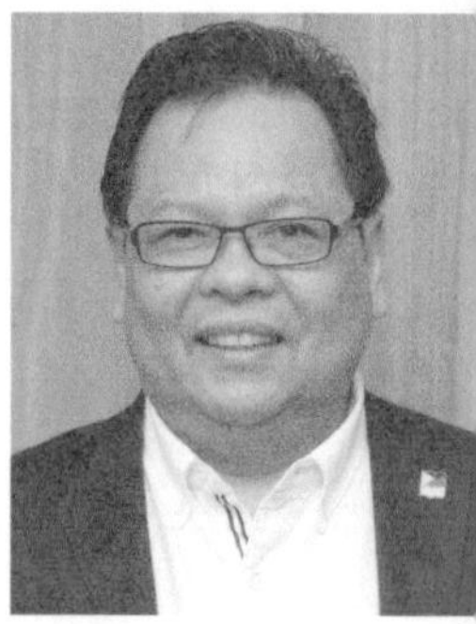
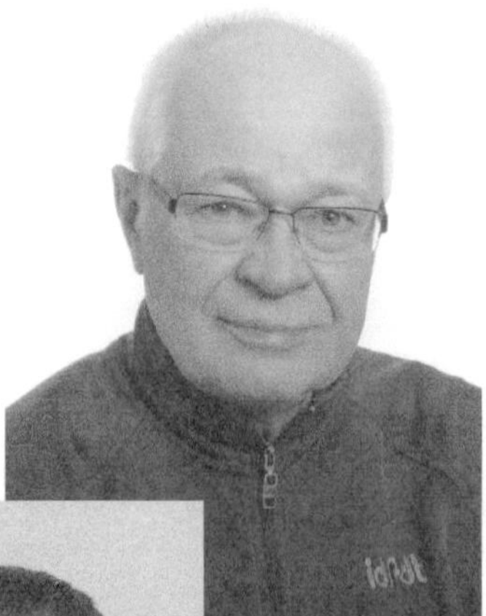
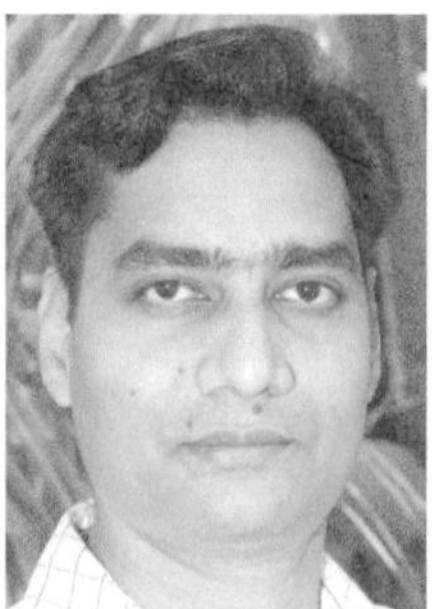
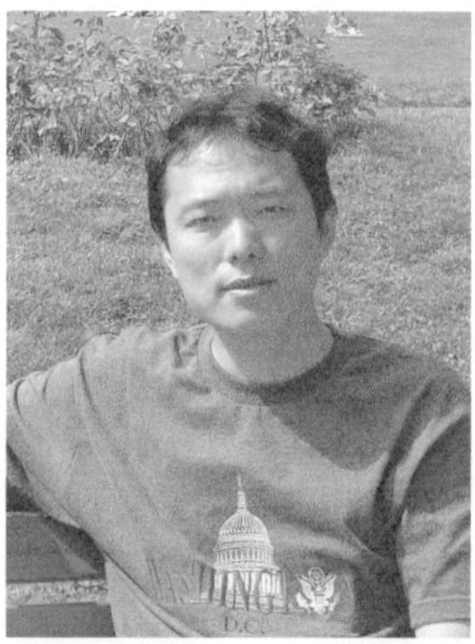
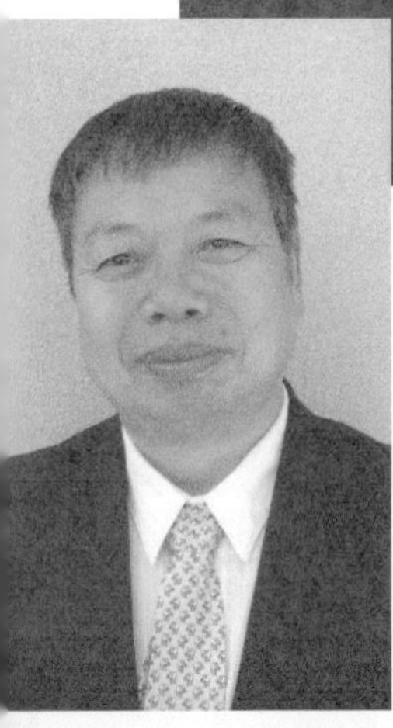
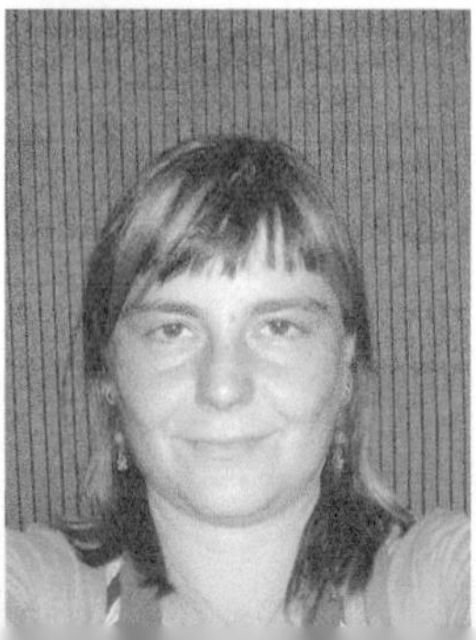

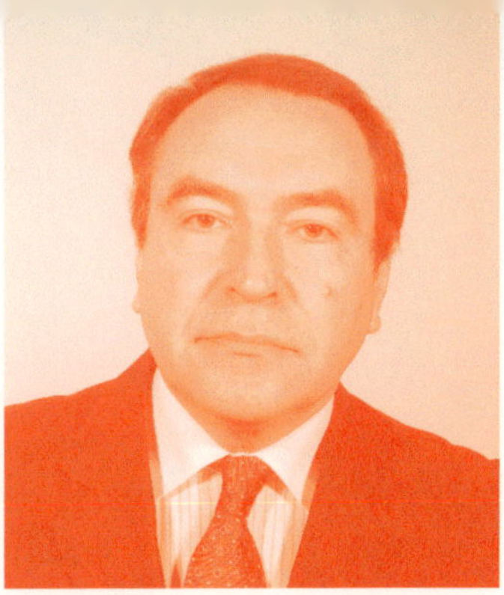
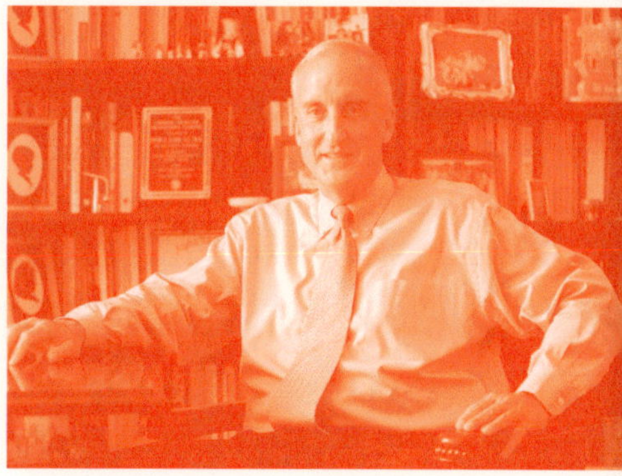
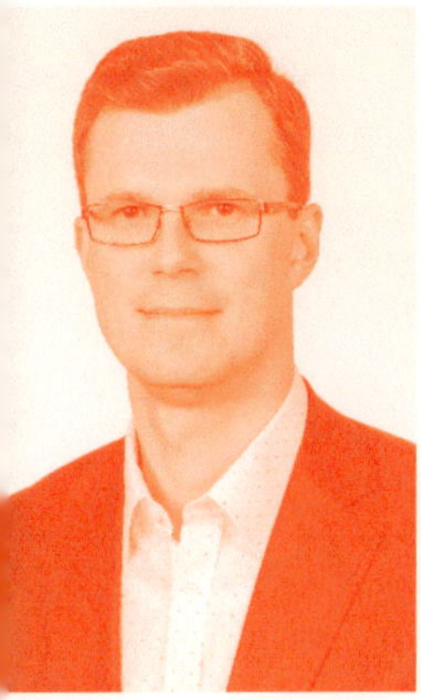
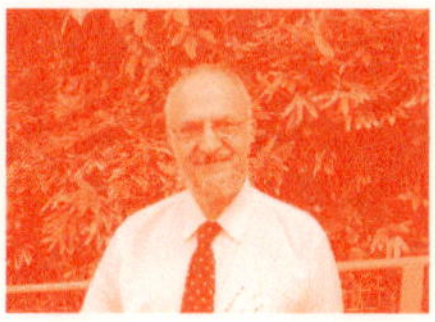
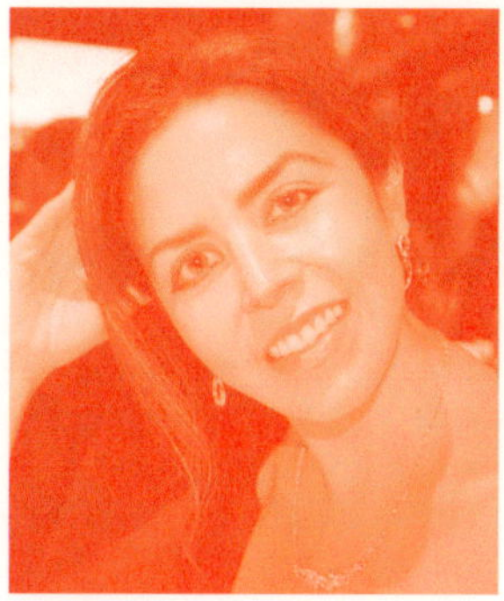

Supporting open minds since 2005

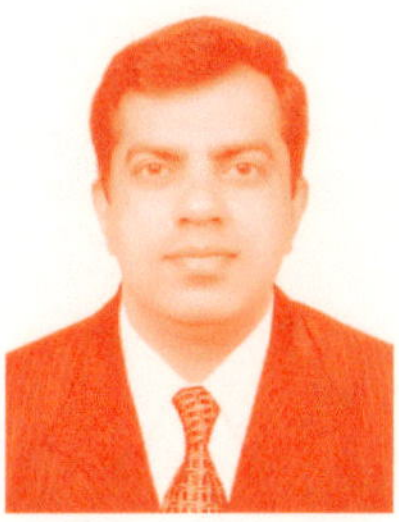
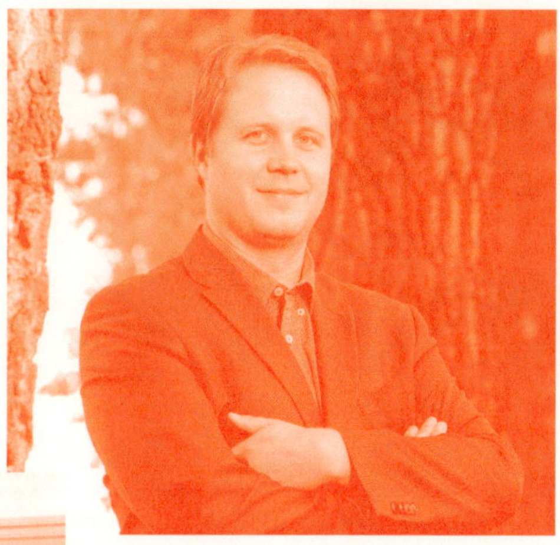
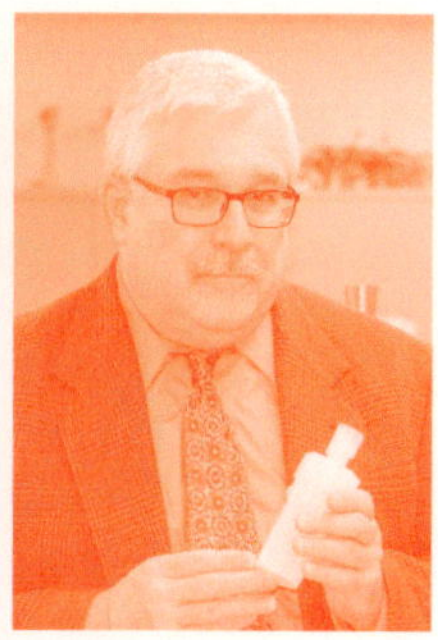
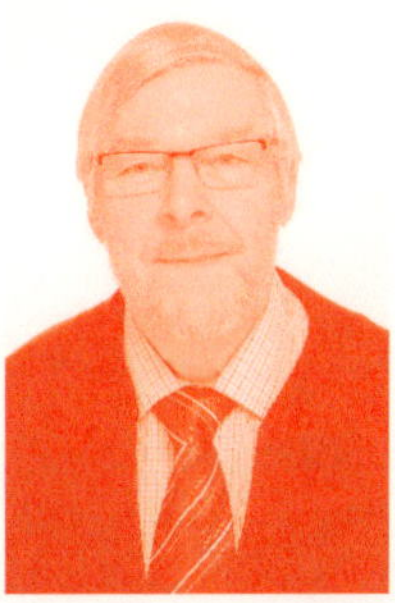
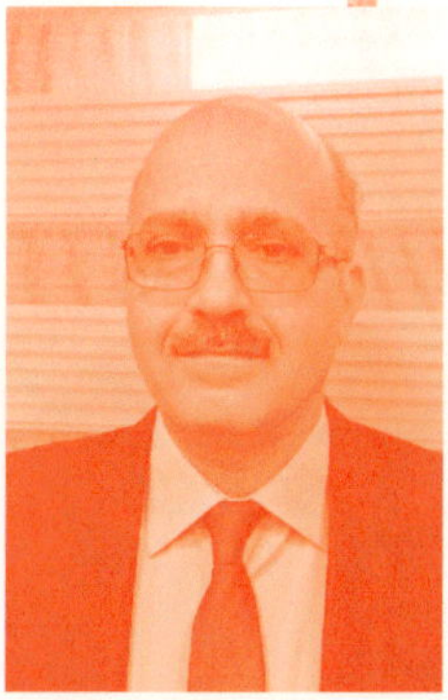
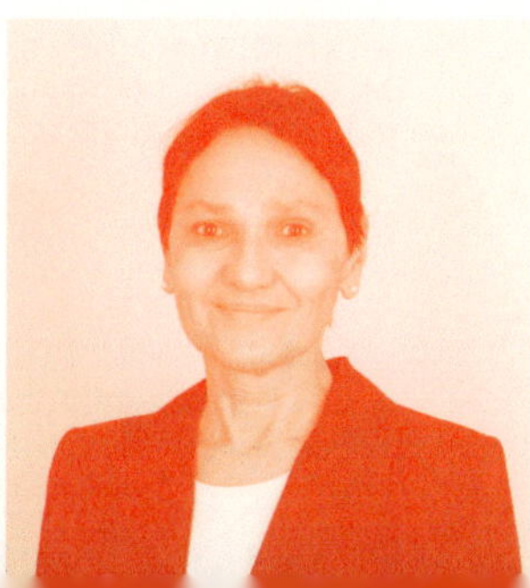
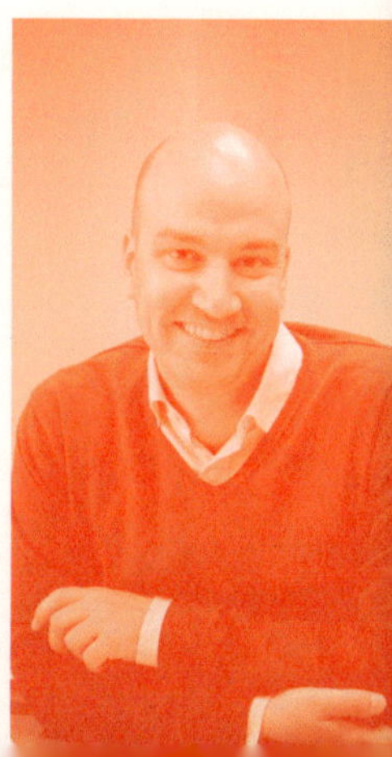

Biomedical Signal and Image Processing
http://dx.doi.org/10.5772/intechopen.87771
Edited by Yongxia Zhou

Part of IntechOpen Book Series: Biomedical Engineering, Volume 10
Book Series Editor: Robert Koprowski

Contributors
Hasna Albandar, Veturia Chiroiu, Ligia Munteanu, Nicoleta Nedelcu, Cristian Rugină, Pablo Revuelta Sanz, María José Lucía Mudas, Tomás Ortiz, José M. Sánchez-Pena, Belen Ruiz-Mezcua, Yousif Mohamed Y. Mohamed Yousif Abdallah, Abdullah Alamoudi, Hasan Kiziltoprak, Kemal Tekin, Dilara Ozkoyuncu, Mustafa Koc, Eduardo Rojas Alvarez

First published in London, United Kingdom, 2021 by IntechOpen
IntechOpen is the global imprint of INTECHOPEN LIMITED, registered in England and Wales, registration number: 11086078, 5 Princes Gate Court, London, SW7 2QJ, United Kingdom
Printed in Croatia

British Library Cataloguing-in-Publication Data
A catalogue record for this book is available from the British Library

Additional hard and PDF copies can be obtained from orders@intechopen.com

Biomedical Signal and Image Processing
Edited by Yongxia Zhou
p. cm.
Print ISBN 978-1-83968-444-9
Online ISBN 978-1-83968-445-6
eBook (PDF) ISBN 978-1-83968-446-3
ISSN 2631-5343

For EU product safety concerns:
IN TECH d.o.o., Prolaz Marije Krucifikse Kozulić 3, 51000 Rijeka, Croatia, info@intechopen.com or visit our website at intechopen.com.

IntechOpen Book Series

Biomedical Engineering

Volume 10

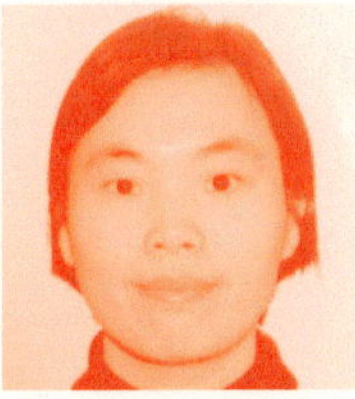

Yongxia Zhou obtained a Ph.D. in Biomedical Imaging from the University of Southern California. Her areas of interest include radiology and neuroscience technology and application. She trained as an imaging scientist at several prestigious institutes including Columbia University, University of Pennsylvania, and the National Institutes of Health (NIH). Her research focuses on multi-modal neuroimaging integration such as MRI/PET and EEG/MEG instrumentation to make the best use of multiple modalities for better interpretation of underlying disease mechanisms. She is the author and editor of more than twelve books for well-known publishers and has published more than 100 papers and abstracts in many reputed international journals and conferences. She has also served as a reviewer and editor for several academic associations.

Editor of Volume 10:
Yongxia Zhou
University of Southern California and Columbia University
Los Angeles, California, USA

Book Series Editor:
Robert Koprowski
University of Silesia, Poland

Scope of the Series

Biomedical engineering is one of the fastest-growing interdisciplinary branches of science and industry. The combination of electronics and computer science with biology and medicine has resulted in improved patient diagnosis, reduced rehabilitation time, and better quality of life. Nowadays, all medical imaging devices, medical instruments, or new laboratory techniques are the result of the cooperation of specialists in various fields. The series of biomedical engineering books covers such areas of knowledge as chemistry, physics, electronics, medicine and biology. This series is intended for doctors, engineers and scientists involved in biomedical engineering or those wanting to start working in this field.

Contents

Preface

Biomedical Signal and Image Processing provides full perspectives of methodological developments, comprehensive modeling, and integration of multiple imaging modalities, as well as various disease applications in the medical imaging field. Methodological developments cover advanced biomedical imaging processing techniques such as image segmentation and registration, image reconstruction and feature selection for classification, tissue deformation simulation, and high-level interpretation and statistical analyses. Multi-modality imaging and integration such as MRI and EEG, perfusion and diffusion, tissue-environment characterization with microscopy, and molecular imaging diagnosis can improve disease detection accuracy and make the best use of each imaging modality to achieve greater spatiotemporal resolution and better illustration of underlying pathophysiological processes. The book provides a thorough review of cutting-edge biomedical imaging techniques and quantitative elucidation of applications in diverse areas and challenging diseases such as neuroscience, chemotherapy, ophthalmology, and stroke. It also provides information on radiation safety in medical imaging. The contents of this volume are of great interest and high significance to the development and generalization of novel biomedical technology and advanced medical research.

The first section of this book covers important perspectives of integrated signal and imaging processing and advanced research. Chapter 1 "Mapping and Timing the (Healthy) Emotional Brain: A Review" outlines EEG and fMRI modalities from background to application with a focus on imaging emotional response of the brain in the neuroscience framework. It outlines via illustrations and examples the importance of spatiotemporal mapping of emotion in healthy brains with different stimuli, EEG for temporal information and fMRI for spatial localization, and integration of EEG/fMRI for simultaneous measuring and comparison. For instance, it elaborates on the detection and functional roles of the initial EEG event-related potential P300 as well as the late positive potential (LPP) in response to emotional stimuli, together with several brain circuits and regions such as the amygdala and fronto-mesolimbic network for neuronal correlates of emotion. Chapter 2 "Modeling of the Flexible Needle Insertion into the Human Liver" provides an accurate and insightful description of integrated molecular imaging diagnosis-based intraoperative needle insertion into the liver for tumor chemotherapy delivery. The chapter fully demonstrates surgery simulation, deformation of the needle and interaction with the liver within the framework of Cosserat elasticity theory, and incorporation of the local rotation and liver force stress. The deformation and tissue interaction problems are formed and solved with the cnoidal wave propagation method. Accurate and quantitative formulas with illustrative figures are strong points of this chapter.

The second section of this book covers the topics of microscopy technologies, utilities, and various applications. Chapter 3 "Confocal Scanning Laser Microscopy in Medicine" elaborates the Confocal Scanning Laser Microscopy (CSLM) technique and advances in several fields. CSLM is a non-invasive imaging method that provides morphological details with high resolution and generates enface images with excellent depth discrimination. The chapter thus describes the principles of CSLM and its application in ophthalmology, including semitransparent tissues and corneal cells as well as nerve and related disease diagnostics such as keratoconus and refractive surgery. It also discusses the method's use in non-ophthalmological areas of medicine such as dentistry. Some ongoing and future developments with relatively novel instrumentation are also introduced in the areas of multi-photon and slit-lamp microscopy technologies as well as optical coherence tomography. Chapter 4 "Cornea Confocal Microscopy: Utilities and Perspectives" summarizes the procedure for performing corneal confocal microscopy, the normal characteristics of the tissue with real images of patients, and potential future applications of the procedure. This technique has extensive applications in corneal dystrophies (keratoconus), refractive surgery, corneal transplantation, infectious keratitis, glaucoma filtration bulla, and diabetes. Microscopy image interpretation with advanced methodologies including intensity normalization, micro-texture quantification, shape characterization, connecting-fiber distribution, the field of view/contrast/resolution, and edge detection are illustrated in various signal processing aspects.

The third section of this book discusses radiation safety issues in imaging processing and stroke applications. Chapter 5 "Occupational Health and Radiation Safety of Radiography Workers" addresses important occupational and radiation safety topics for health workers, especially radiologists. Some critical concerns and diseases such as radiation and nosocomial and occupational infection are covered in detail. The chapter summarizes several techniques for handling contamination including isolation, precautions, and surgery. Radiation protection for preventing the harmful effects of ionizing radiation exposure is critical and could benefit both physicians and patients. Chapter 6 "Characterization of Brain Stroke Using Image and Signal Processing Techniques" reviews characterizations of brain stroke using image and signal processing techniques. It outlines stroke classification, signs and symptoms, and causes. It also examines the diagnosis of stroke with multiple imaging techniques including MRI and CT, together with empirical post-processing methods such as segmentation and morphological transformation. Finally, it compares subtypes of stroke based on distinct imaging features for better interpretation and diagnosis.

Yongxia Zhou, Ph.D.
Imaging Scientist,
University of Southern California and Columbia University,
Los Angeles, California, USA

Section 1

Integrated Signal and Imaging Processing

Chapter 1

Mapping and Timing the (Healthy) Emotional Brain: A Review

Pablo Revuelta Sanz, María José Lucía Mulas, Tomás Ortiz, José M. Sánchez Pena and Belén Ruiz-Mezcua

Abstract

The study of the emotional processing in the brain began from a psychological point of view in the last decades of the 19th century. However, since the discovery of the electrical background of mental activity around 1930, a new scientific way of observing and measuring the functioning of the living brain has opened up. In addition, Functional Magnetic Resonance Imaging (fMRI) has given neuroscientists a (literally) deeper instrument to perform such measurements. With all this technological background, the last decades have produced an important amount of information about how the brain works. In this chapter, we review the latest results on the emotional response of the brain, a growing field in neuroscience.

Keywords: brain, EEG, fMRI, emotions, stimuli, neuroscience

1. Introduction

The study of emotions deals with the physiological and psychological correlates of subjective experiences that are evident to conscious human beings. Emotions are present and influence our lives and even our perception of reality, making the scientific approach to their study, which has only begun in relatively recent decades, very difficult.

According to [1], the pseudoscience of phrenology brought the critical idea of the physical distribution of psychological functions in the brain, opening the door to modern neuroscience that has largely corroborated this assumption.

It is widely assumed that emotions are the subjective representations of naturally evolved primarily neural circuits and functions that helped surviving since the very first complex animals [2, 3]. This has two main consequences: on the one hand, the physical localization of emotional circuits is hidden in the ancient brain (the limbic system, the amygdalae, and other inner regions). On the other hand, these regions are largely connected to more developed areas, such as the cortex or the cerebellum. Therefore, not only should external stimuli trigger automatic motor responses, but cognitive information can be critical as well as a "brake" on these autonomous reactions (implemented in the cerebellum) and can produce more flexible and adaptive responses.

Although much research in this field focuses on damaged brains, this review covers the healthy brain that responds to emotional stimuli under laboratory conditions.

1.1 History

The connection between the physical processes of the brain and its biomarkers has been assumed since the late 19th century [4].

In 1929, German psychiatrist Hans Berger developed the novel method of Electro-Encephalography (EEG), opening a disruptive and scientific way of studying the processes of the living brain. Although a vast and unexplored field was opened, the first results using EEG to measure emotions did not occur until the 1960s [5]. However, interest in emotional studies still had to wait some years, till the mid-70s' when some researches began to appear [6, 7].

Since then, the same basic experimental setup has been replicated in research until today: a subject connected to the EEG, or to new tomography technologies (as in [8]), is exposed to different stimuli while his brain activity is recorded.

Figure 1 shows the historic timeline developing this research field.

Positron Emission Tomography (PET) and Magnetic Resonance Imaging (MRI), two new techniques to access information inside the brain, and not only at scalp level, were developed in 1975 and 1979 respectively, and began to yield significant results in the 1980s (see, for example, [10]).

1.2 Brain atlases and areas' references

The brain began to be mapped according to its anatomical differences in 1909 by Brodmann [11], who defined 52 regions that modern neuroscience considers extraordinarily accurate for those years. In fact, today most neuroscientific works still provide Brodmann's nomenclature to specify the areas of activation.

However, it has been shown that it is not precise enough to evaluate some functional characteristics of the brain, so the Montreal Neurological Institute proposed in the 1990s a more modern division of the human brain [12], with 1 mm^3 templates organized in a system of coordinates (X, Y, Z). Today, this brain atlas is considered to be a standard.

The main regions in the brain are depicted in the **Figure 2**.

1.3 Emotional maps

Emotions are subjective feelings, but they must be quantified in some way to allow a methodical study. Since the 1980s, there have been two main approaches in the field of emotion research: the categorical approach and the dimensional approach.

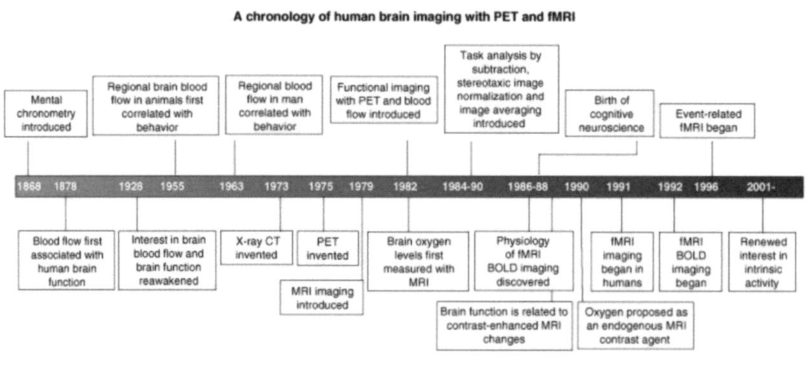

Figure 1.
A chronology of major events associated with the development of human brain imaging, from [9], adapted with permission.

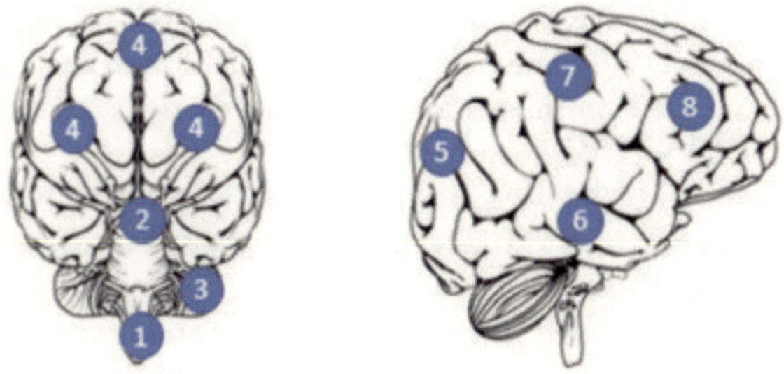

Figure 2.
Basic brain anatomy. 1: Brain stem. 2: Limbic system. 3: Cerebellum. 4: Cerebrum. 5: Occipital lobe. 6: Temporal lobe. 7: Parietal lobe. 8: Frontal lobe.

The dimensional approach considers that emotions are organized along a few psychological dimensions. Step by step, a consensus was established on the representation of emotions around a two-dimensional plane, shown in **Figure 3**.

The debate about the separation of the emotional features of valence and arousal flows over the correlation of these two variables. Barret, for example, found weak correlation between them [14], and Lang supports this idea, inferring that some neural circuits are similarly engaged by motivationally relevant cues independently of the valence, while there may be some other hedonic circuits to discriminate valence [3, 15]. However, other researchers have found contradictory results [16], specifically with respect to valence and arousal of negative stimuli.

This paradigm presents another issue since Miller's studies [17]. It seems that there is a distortion in the linearity of this space: a negativity bias (for equal amount of positive or negative stimulus, the negative one produces higher responses) and a positive offset (in neutral scenarios, there is a predisposition to appetitive responses).

Combinations of different scales have been used to provide representational spaces with more dimensions and, allegedly, higher accuracy [16]. Examples of these rating scales are the Bivariate Evaluation and Ambivalent Measures (BEAM), described in [18] and the three-dimensional space proposed in [19], which distinguishes between tension arousal and energy arousal.

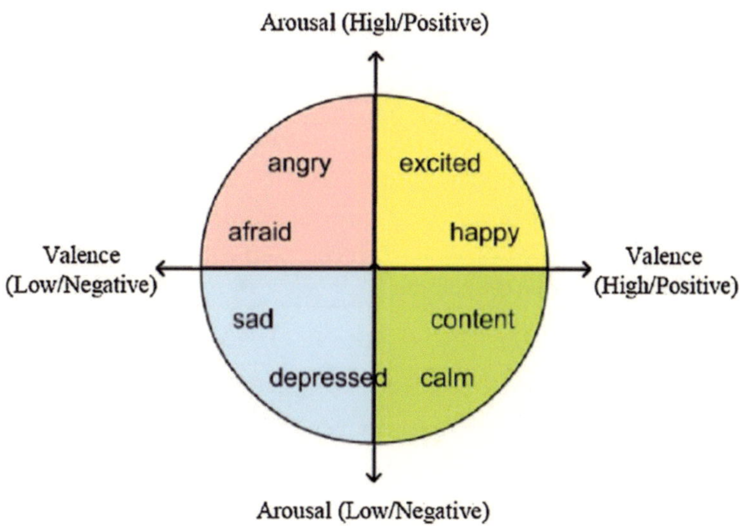

Figure 3.
Emotional map from [13], adapted with permission.

As an example of categorical approach, we can find the Self-Assessment Manikin (SAM): SAM is a non-verbal pictorial assessment technique that directly measures the valence, arousal, and dominance associated with a person's affective reaction to a wide variety of stimuli [20].

There is an important body of evidence supporting cross-cultural stability in the perception of emotions [21, 22], and the pleasant-unpleasant dimension seems to exists in all cultures [23]. Ekman considers a few categories of innate and universal emotions (happiness, sadness, anger, fear and disgust) from which all other emotions can be derived [24]. The categorical approach that considers some discrete emotional maps related to basic adaptive problems, has been shown to be cross-cultural or even cross-species (for a review, please refer to [25]).

1.4 Emotional stimuli

As stated in the History section, the setup of most of neuroscientific experiments involves stimuli to elicit emotions (or any other response) in the subject under study.

In addition, different stimuli trigger different and specific areas of the brain, so the choice of stimuli is crucial for the information expected to be retrieved from the experiment.

We will present the most used ones and some points about their effectiveness.

1.4.1 Emotion elicitation techniques

Out of a total of 248 articles, al-Nafjan gathers the type of stimulus used in **Table 1**.

Why using images?

Psychologists have already shown that images have strong effects on the emotions of human beings [16]. An important result found in the literature states that simple images generate better emotional responses than complex scenes [3, 27].

Please refer to [28] for a deeper review.

Why using music?

The role of music in producing emotional responses is widely accepted and is one of its defining features [29]. Moreover, this has been proven to be cross-cultural [30, 31], making it a very stable and reliable way to provoke emotions in subjects.

When using audio-visual stimuli, it is important to take into account the predominance of image over sound [32], in case of ambiguity or emotional conflict.

Technique	Number of Articles	Domain (Medical, Non-Medical)
Visual-based elicitation using images	88	26%, 73.9%
Prepared task	43	25.6%, 47.4%
Audio-visual elicitation using short film video clips	38	18.4%, 81.6%
Audio-based elicitation using music	29	17.2%, 82.8%
Multiple techniques	19	26.3%, 73.9%
Other	17	11.7%, 88.2%
Imagination techniques/memory recall	10	20%, 80%
Social interactions	4	25%, 75%

Table 1.
Emotional stimuli used according to their nature, from [26].

DOI: http://dx.doi.org/10.5772/intechopen.95574

Why using words?

It is well known that the brain dedicates exclusive resources, organized hierarchically, to word and language processing, such as the areas of Broca and Wernicke, which demonstrates their importance in evolution and survival. It has subsequently been found that words and language stimuli function as emotional triggers [33, 34].

Others

Among the "other" stimuli in **Table 1**, researchers have used olfactory [35, 36] or food [37] stimulation, for example.

1.4.2 Databases

To ease the replication, comparison and contrast of theories and results, many research institutions and authors have developed databases with normalized emotional stimuli, which are publicly available. They have labeled stimuli according to different paradigms, and they have been tested. Some of the most used ones are the following:

- Surrey Audio-Visual Expressed Emotion (SAVEE) Database: Audio-visual clips with male actors in different emotions [38].

- International Affective Picture System (IAPS): This database offers a "large set of standardized, emotionally-evocative, internationally-accessible, color photographs that includes contents across a wide range of semantic categories" [39].

- International Affective Digital Sounds (IADS): The same institution and researchers have published the International Affective Digitized Sound system (IADS), with similar structure, labeling and testing parameters [40].

- Affective Norms for English Words (ANEW): The word-based version of the previous couple of databases [41].

- Affective Norms for English Text (ANET): In the case of using text extracts, this database "provides normative ratings of emotion (pleasure, arousal, dominance) for a large set of brief texts in the English language for use in experimental investigations of emotion and attention" [42].

- The Ryerson Audio-Visual Database of Emotional Speech and Song (RAVDESS): This is a multimodal database of emotional speech and songs, labeled following a discrete emotional space, with neutral stimuli included [43].

- The Montreal Affective Voices (MAV) consist of a set of short vocal interjections expressing anger, disgust, fear, pain, sadness, surprise, happiness, sensual pleasure, and neutrality [44].

As we have seen, the databases cover language, images, sounds and combinations thereof.

2. Methods

Nowadays, almost all neuroscientific studies and findings are based on two non-invasive, biomarkers-free technologies: Electroencephalography (EEG) and functional Magnetic Resonance Imaging (fMRI).

2.1 EEG

The EEG is based on the evidence that massive clusters of neurons fire at the same time when they work synchronized, producing tiny voltage changes around them (in the range of millivolts to microvolts). The EEG can be measured directly on the surface of the brain surface and scalp. In both cases, the system has the following elements:

- Electrodes: conductive elements sensitive to voltage variations.
- Amplifier: low-noise, band-filtered amplifier to scale the small voltage measured.
- Register: Analog or (nowadays) digital recording of the transformed signals, together with time stamps, position information and other contextual information.

Important advantages of this technique are its setup (some equipment is portable) and its price (actually, the cheapest of the techniques exposed here). In the scalp version, it is non-invasive and very safe for the subject.

The main advantage of this technique is the time resolution, around the millisecond, which measures very rapid changes in scalp potentials. Because of this, only the EEG technique allows phase measurements, synchronization computations, spectral analysis, or other time-related processing.

In the EEG, the first representational information found was the so-called Event-Related Potentials (ERPs), signals produced as a reaction to a stimulus, typically within a few hundred milliseconds to several seconds. These signals have proven to be stable between users and experiments, and some of them, as the P300 (positive peak 300 ms after stimulus onset), are universally known and used.

The EEG allows frequency analysis, and its signals can be transformed into bands. The spectral power (also called Power Spectral Density -PSD-), i.e., the amount of energy in each band-, can be used to obtain important information from the raw EEG data.

Since 1977 [45], researchers have proposed a new approach, combining the ERPs and the bands, called Event-Related Synchronization (ERS) and Desynchronization (ERD), to measure instantaneous responses to stimuli in specific bands, as shown in **Figure 4**.

The main counterparts of this technique are the volume conductance effect that makes it difficult to locate internal potential sources [47], and the limitation of recording only signals on the surface of the brain (if no electrodes are placed inside the brain), which also limits the measurement of internal sources. To partially address this limitation, some novel techniques recreate inner sources from their fingerprint on the scalp voltage through complex algorithms, such as the Low Resolution Electromagnetic Tomography (LORETA) first proposed in [48], and other "reverse problem methods" summarized in [49, 50].

In addition, EEG registers suffer from artifacts (from electrical power networks, lighting, muscle movements ...) that must be removed or filtered out before the recordings can be interpreted. Although some automatic approaches have been proposed, this is a craft task that many researchers still perform manually. Another source of noise is the impedance of the electrodes (as they are transductors between the scalp and the wires), which must be kept low enough to accurately measure extremely low scalp voltages, typically below 50 Ω. This requires the application of a conductive gel, cleaning with electrodes with alcohol, washing the hair before the experiment, etc.

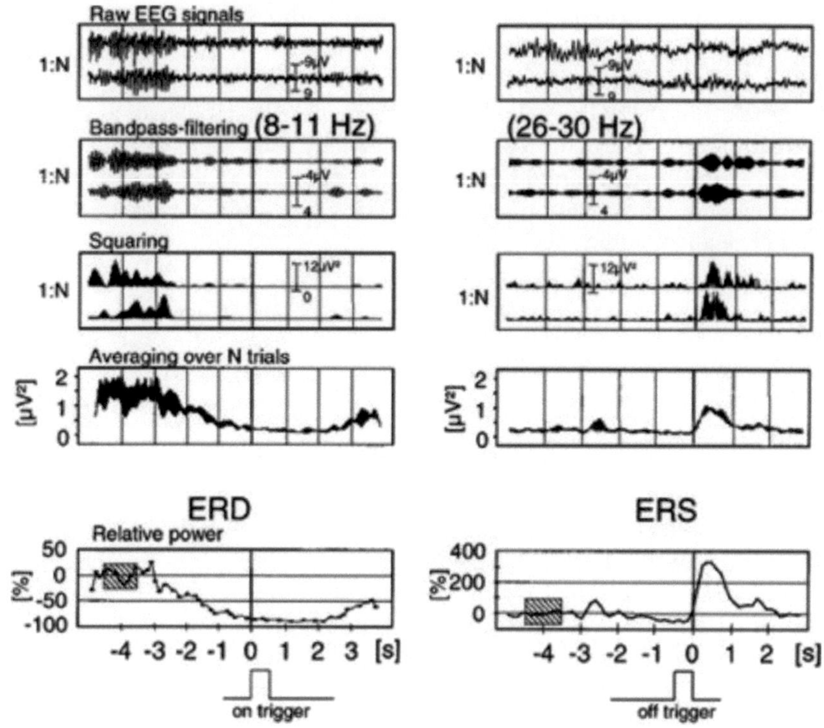

Figure 4.
ERD/ERS detection, from [46], adapted with permission.

Finally, the EEG system, as a voltage recorder, needs a reference. This does not change the relative voltage distribution on the scalp, but depending on the choice, it can lead to different absolute measures.

Another important process of standardization of EEG measurements has been the definition of electrode positions, which must be constant between studies to allow replication and falsifiability. Depending on the number of electrodes, different standard configurations are defined, the most used being, in the case of 32, the 10–20 International configuration of **Figure 5**.

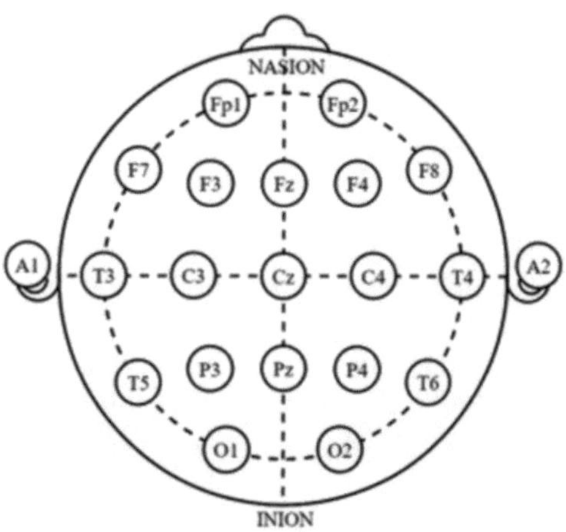

Figure 5.
The 10–20 international EEG configuration.

The names and positions of the electrodes are defined in this standard and applied elsewhere. For a larger number of electrodes some other standards can be found (see, for example, [51]).

The correlation of EEG signals with emotions is well established, as stated in [26]: " We found that the majority of the 130 articles used event-related potentials, whereas 48 articles used Frontal EEG asymmetry in their analysis, six articles used event-related desynchronization/synchronization, and four articles used steady-state visually evoked potentials".

2.2 fRMI

fMRI began in the 1980s, and soon produced extremely novel results. fMRI measures differential activations of brain regions [52] according to de-oxy-hemoglobin distribution.

fMRI requires a massive magnet (typically around a few tesla), which makes the setup extremely space demanding and expensive. Besides, it cannot be used with metallic components (nor implanted in the subject's body) so the presentation of the stimuli must be deviated with reflective screens, remote speakers, etc.

The temporal resolution of fMRI is poor, in the range of seconds, which makes it useless to record rapid changes or reactions to the stimuli. However, the main positive aspect is the spatial resolution and the real three-dimensionality of the recording, which generates a map of voxels (volumetric units of information) of very few mm^3 if a high temporal resolution is not needed (in fact there is a trade-off between these two parameters; for example, for a voxel size of $3x3x5mm^3$, the sampling rate falls to about 2 s [53]). Unlike the EEG registering technique, fMRI has the difficulty of mapping different brains (of different participants) in a canonical brain in which the activations and regions can be represented. This forces a spatial transformation to standard geometries that implies loses in spatial resolution [53].

The functionality of the MRI is given, among others, by the Blood Oxygen Level Dependent (BOLD) imaging, which measures differences in oxygenated blood flowing through the brain (since oxy-hemoglobin and de-oxy-hemoglobin have different magnetic susceptibility), correlated with neural activation.

BOLD techniques have the temporal limitations of the physiological processes on which they are based (see [53] for more details). In most studies, fMRI data are statistically processed to generate a meaningful representation of changes, in so-called Statistical Parametric Maps (SPM), yielding to images as that shown in **Figure 6**.

2.3 Simultaneous measuring and comparison

Since both EEG and fRMI are based on related physiological processes, it is easy to find correlations between them.

These two non-invasive techniques for exploring the interior of the living brain are not mutually exclusive, and both have advantages and disadvantages. Therefore, both are used in neuroscience research today.

Table 2 summarizes the main characteristics of each one.

In 1996, Gerloff and others [54] combined fMRI and EEG for the first time to evaluate the co-registration of both techniques applied to the primary motor cortex and the sensory cortex.

Over the past decade, several studies using both techniques have been proposed to, among other, find new large-scale brain networks [55], examine some specific networks [56–58] or even provide neurofeedback to assist in the regulation of some circuits [59].

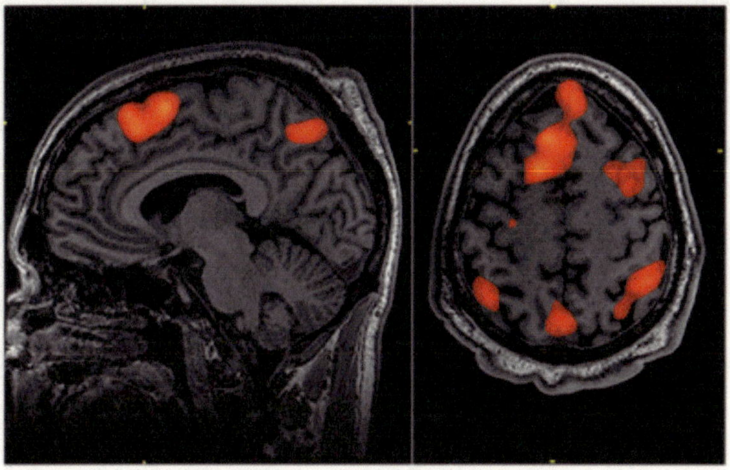

Figure 6.
SPM in which the color of pixels is representative of its p-value and, thus, the statistical significance of its activation or deactivation when two or more tasks are compared. From G.Konstantina, CC BY-SA 4.0, via Wikimedia commons.

Technique	Temporal Resolution	Spatial Resolution	Portability
EEG	High	Low	Mid
fMRI	Low	High	Low

Table 2.
Features comparison between EEG and fMRI.

Babayan et al. [60] have recently published a large database with combined EEG and fMRI data from 227 healthy participants.

Unfortunately, the joint use of both techniques has its drawbacks: the signal-to-noise ratio (SNR) can be degraded [61] and interferential artifacts can be generated, as shown in [62].

For more in-depth in brain data imaging, please refer to the handbook [63].

3. Measuring emotions

The neuronal correlates of emotions present features and effects in various dimensions that interact in the living brain.

To help understand the results collected in the scientific literature on emotions, we will divide the findings into different categories, although they are mixed and sometimes inseparable.

3.1 Timing

Studies dealing with the temporal signals created by the emotional processing are, most of the time, based on EEG recordings. The reason is, as explained, the temporal resolution of this technique.

Typically, the measurement of an EEG signal follows the scheme of **Figure 7**.

When recording the brain's reaction to stimuli, it is important to define a control group or baseline with which to compare activations or deactivations. Koelstra [65] proposes 5 seconds prior to stimuli as such a baseline.

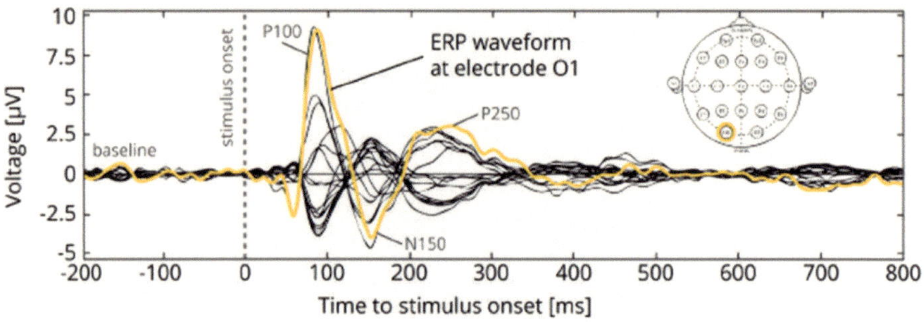

Figure 7.
Typical EEG signal during a stimulus-based experiment, from [64], adapted with permission.

What happens in the reference period is not uninteresting when emotions are studied from a neuroscientific approach. It has been proven that if in this period the index of asymmetry (the difference in the global activation in each hemisphere, calculated as the left over the right) is high, the subject will present a bias towards positive stimuli, and vice versa as far as fear is concerned [66].

After the stimulus onset, Wei defines a time range of [0.5–4] s as the temporal space in which emotional signals appear [13]. This period has been divided by some authors into three sections: Early [400–1100] ms, Middle [1000-3000] ms, Late [3000–5000] ms [32].

For example, it is widely established that a high positive ERP, in the range of 200–300 ms, widely known as P300, is elicited by emotional stimuli (such as emotional words) compared to neutral ones [67–71]. This ERP appears in the occipital-temporal regions with an arousal-related amplitude (independent of the valence) compared to neutral stimuli [72].

As already mentioned, the emotional response is mediated or modulated by different neural systems. The P300 has proven to be a modulator of emotional processing regardless of valence when presenting emotional versus neutral pictures [5, 67, 73–75]. These effects were seen in both pleasant and unpleasant pictures [5, 75, 76].

One of the most stable and reliable neural signatures of emotional processing is the so-called Late Positive Potential (LPP), which appears after 1 second of the stimulus presentation, and can be traced for up to 6 seconds in the central-parietal region [77].

It has been shown that LPP appears with both emotional pictures or words, with an amplitude that depends on the arousal intensity [67, 70, 71], being higher in emotional (both positive and negatives) images compared to neutral ones [78] and not habit-forming [67, 79, 80], although it may decrease somewhat with repetition [15]. Another interesting feature of this signal is its ability to appear with very short exposures to visual stimuli (down to 25 ms) [3].

The LPP is independent of the characteristics of the stimuli as realism/symbolism, complexity/simplicity, etc. [27, 67] and therefore very reliable: "The late positive potential evoked by picture stimuli is a reliable, replicable index of their motivational relevance" [3], correlated with the self-reported arousal [3].

For all these reasons, the LPP has been labeled as the "motivational significance" of a stimulus [81].

The LPP has been localized in the central-parietal region, but also in the secondary visual processing sites in the lateral occipital cortex [82] with visual stimuli.

Summarizing the findings of time-analysis of EEG signals correlated with emotional processing, we can say that the P300 and LPP track emotional processes [78]. There is a golden rule that says that valence is processed before arousal [83], since it has been shown that the early ERP components are correlated with valence [28, 84]. In contrast, the long-term ERP components are correlated with the arousal [85–87].

Hajcak et al. [67] illustrate the temporal and spatial evolution of the different signals.

3.2 Mapping

The fMRI has shown the processing cores in the inner regions of the brain, such as the limbic system. In terms of arousal, it was found that the area of greatest response in the brain is the amygdalae, a couple of little clusters of nuclei belonging to the limbic system in the temporal lobes, on the internal part of the brain. Regarding the role of the amygdalae in emotional processing, survival instincts, memory, etc. Lang et al. found that this area responds to the intensity of emotional stimuli, and has a central role in enhancing sympathetic reactivity to such stimuli [15]. But the amygdalae do not react independently of the valence of the stimuli: the preferred stimuli selectively activated the right amygdala, in relation to aversive ones in some experiments [88, 89].

Valence has also been correlated with specific limbic neural circuits closely connected to the amygdalae: the mesolimbic reward system, in which the nucleus accumbens (NAc) is particularly relevant in the processing of reward and pleasure evoking stimuli (the reward, motivation and addiction circuits) [90, 91]. Another study extends this list of central processing centers to the Ventral Tegmental Area (VTA) and the hypothalamus, working together as a tripartite network that manages the responses to the emotional aspects of music [92]. Another reward network component is the ventral striatum, which, along with the cingulate cortex, has also shown correlations with the arousal of positive emotions when listening to music [93, 94].

The relation between the mesolimbic networks and some frontal regions (as the Orbito-Frontal Cortex (OFC) and the Interior Frontal Cortex (IFC)), more in charge of cognitive processing, has led some researchers to establish a close relationship between "affective" and "cognitive" processing involved in music listening [92]. Another hypothesis is that the interactions between the OFC and the NAc may be related to the control of emotions [95].

Overall, although it belongs to the cognitive cortex, the role of the OFC in the emotional processing is beyond doubt, and is supported by many studies dealing with music [32, 92, 96, 97], images [98, 99] or decisions [95]. Close to the OFC, the IFC has also been considered relevant, producing a bilateral activation when listening to music, according to [92].

Other important cortex cores for emotional processing are the parietal and temporal areas. The centro-parietal area has shown an activation proportional to the arousal of emotional pictures in the first moments (in a range of 300 to 700 ms) [3, 92]. Positive centro-parietal signals [300–6000 ms] have shown valence independence [3]. Furthermore, the link between the frontal and right parieto-temporal areas with the arousal of a stimulus has been also established [100].

It is worth mentioning the anterior insula, belonging to the temporal lobe, which has been thoroughly studied and defined as a relay between the limbic (specifically the human mirror neuron system) and the motor system (in the cortex) [31, 101], and may be the physiological support for subjective states, like pain, hunger, heart rate perception or emotional awareness [102–104].

Early lateralization has been found to be correlated with the valence of sounds [32], and this effect does not exist with neutral sounds. One of the first findings in this field is due to Schwartz [7], who found a lateralization in the brain activity.

Back to the surface of the cortex, there are areas specially engaged in emotional processing, measured with both EEG and fMRI.

In the first case, there is a discussion about which electrodes are the most representative of the undergoing emotional processes. For example, we can find the work of Wei et al., who proposes moving from F1, F2, T3 and T4 to F1, F2, F7 and F8 respectively (shifting the registering area from bilateral front-temporal to pre-frontal medial areas), obtaining much better predictions [13]. This change is also proposed independently (and partially) by Lin et al., stating that fronto-central electrodes are specially relevant when measuring theta asymmetry (F7-F8 and FC3-FC4) as a correlate of arousal [105].

By focusing on synchronizations between different areas, it has been found that there is a phase synchronization between frontal and right temporo-parietal areas depending on the valence and the energetic arousal [106]. In another study [107], a beta-band synchronization was found between the pre-frontal and posterior areas when observing high-arousal images. Finally, unpleasant images caused a phase synchronization in the gamma band according to [108]. Please refer to [109] for further details about synchronization.

We have shown the interactions of the limbic system with the cognitive areas of the brain, in relation to images, sounds or decisions. But we have also found some interactions with other unrelated areas, mainly the motor areas, when empathy in involved. It seems that in the processing of emotions, many different and specialized areas need to interact to account for such a subjective experience. This cross modality has been studied in depth. For example, [32] shows that emotional sounds modulate visual primary cortex (P1). In the same region, relationships have been found between emotional processing cores and visuo-spatial and visuo-motor regions [110], or even premotor regions including the intra-parietal sulcus and the ventral premotor cortex [111]. The ventral premotor and the posterior parietal cortex were elicited during the observation of Classical and Renaissance sculptures suggesting, as Di Dio state, "motor resonance congruent with the implied movements portrayed in the sculptures." [88].

For a final summary, please refer to **Table 1** in [87], which provides a detailed review of the EEG spatial correlates of emotions.

4. Final considerations and conclusions

It has been shown how the way we react to emotional situations depends on very different and scattered areas in the brain. Both initial reactions and the later dependencies lay on different systems [112]. Reward calculation and empathy have been identified as being involved in fear or appetite reactions, and are also the most primitive, but they interact with more evolved areas of the cortex that deal with visual and auditory processing, decision making and even motor activation.

Many aspects of the emotional brain remain open. For instance, global or synchronized processing networks beyond the cortical surface have yet to be described, as the limitations of fMRI and non-invasive EEG do not allow this unknown field to be addressed.

Furthermore, it is not clear whether and how gender affects emotional processing. Although responses to musical stimuli, recorded with EEG, have shown no significant gender differences in brain frontal regions [100], gender differences have been observed during verbal learning tasks [113], in emotional networks in adolescents [114] and with esthetic stimuli producing bilateral parietal activation in women, but lateralized in men [115].

Other limitations are due to the stimuli used. Real life involves interaction with various external and internal sources of information that modulate our feelings, and laboratory conditions barely address such complex situations.

This branch of neuroscience is not new (compared to neuroscience itself), but still presents many open doors to be explored.

The way emotions mobilize resources in the brain seems to be large and deep, and many other functions (such as memory) depend on it, showing their pre-eminent position to survive and behave in human (and many other animals') life.

Author details

Pablo Revuelta Sanz[1*], María José Lucía Mulas[2], Tomás Ortiz[3], José M. Sánchez Pena[2] and Belén Ruiz-Mezcua[2]

1 Oviedo University, Gijón, Spain

2 Spanish Center for Captioning and Audiodescription (CESyA), Leganés, Spain

3 Complutense University, Madrid, Spain

*Address all correspondence to: revueltapablo@uniovi.es

References

[1] A. Damasio, "Descartes Error And The Future Of Human Life," *Scientific American,* vol. 271, no. 4, pp. 144-144, Oct 1994, 1994.

[2] N. Frijda, "The Current Status Of Emotion Theory," *Bulletin of the British Psychological Society,* vol. 39, pp. A75-A75, May 1986, 1986.

[3] P. Lang, and M. Bradley, "Emotion and the motivational brain," *Biological Psychology,* vol. 84, no. 3, pp. 437-450, JUL 2010, 2010.

[4] C. S. Roy, and C. S. Sherrington, "On the Regulation of the Blood-supply of the Brain," *J. Physiol.,* vol. Jan. 11, no. 1-2, pp. 85-158.17., 1890.

[5] K. Lifshitz, "The Averaged Evoked Cortical Response To Complex Visual Stimuli," *Psychophysiology,* vol. 3, no. 1, pp. 55-68, 1966.

[6] Z. Drohocki, "Effect Of Emotion On Amplitude Spectrogram Of EEG," *Electroencephalography and Clinical Neurophysiology,* vol. 36, no. 4, pp. 426-426, 1974, 1974.

[7] G. Schwartz, R. Davidson, And F. Maer, "Right Hemisphere Lateralization For Emotion In Human Brain - Interactions With Cognition," *Science,* vol. 190, no. 4211, pp. 286-288, 1975, 1975.

[8] S. Petersen, P. Fox, M. Posner, M. Mintun, And M. Raichle, "Positron Emission Tomographic Studies Of The Cortical Anatomy Of Single-Word Processing," *Nature,* vol. 331, no. 6157, pp. 585-589, Feb 18 1988, 1988.

[9] M. Raichle, "A brief history of human brain mapping," *Trends in Neurosciences,* vol. 32, no. 2, pp. 118-126, FEB 2009, 2009.

[10] G. Bradac, W. Schorner, A. Bender, And *R. Felix*, "MRI (NMR) IN THE Diagnosis Of Brain-Stem Tumors," *Neuroradiology,* vol. 27, no. 3, pp. 208-213, 1985, 1985.

[11] K. Brodmann, *Vergleichende Lokalisationslehre der Großhirnrinde : in ihren Prinzipien dargestellt auf Grund des Zellenbaues*, Leipzig: Barth, 1909.

[12] A. Evans, M. Kamber, D. Collins, D. Macdonald, S. Shorvon, F. Andermann, G. Bydder, H. Stefan, And D. Fish, "An MRI-Based Probabilistic Atlas Of Neuroanatomy," *Magnetic Resonance Scanning and Epilepsy,* vol. 264, pp. 263-274, 1994, 1994.

[13] Y. Wei, Y. Wu, and J. Tudor, "A real-time wearable emotion detection headband based on EEG measurement," *Sensors and Actuators a-Physical,* vol. 263, pp. 614-621, AUG 15 2017, 2017.

[14] L. Barrett, and J. Russell, "Independence and bipolarity in the structure of current affect," *Journal of Personality and Social Psychology,* vol. 74, no. 4, pp. 967-984, Apr 1998, 1998.

[15] P. Lang, M. Bradley, B. Cuthbert, R. Simons, and M. Balaban, "Motivated attention: Affect, activation, and action," *Attention and Orienting: Sensory and Motivational Processes*, pp. 97-135, 1997, 1997.

[16] T. Ito, J. Cacioppo, and P. Lang, "Eliciting affect using the international affective picture system: Trajectories through evaluative space," *Personality and Social Psychology Bulletin,* vol. 24, no. 8, pp. 855-879, AUG 1998, 1998.

[17] N. E. Miller, "Liberalization of the basic S-R concepts: Extensions to conflict behavior, motivation and social learning," *Psychology: a study of a science*, S. Kock, ed., pp. 198-292, New York: McGraw-Hill, 1959.

[18] J. T. Cacioppo, W. L. Gardner, and G. G. Bernston, "Attitudes and

evaluative space: Beyond bipolar conceptualizations and measures," *Personality and Social Psychology Review,* vol. 1, pp. 3-25, 1997.

[19] U. Schimmack, and A. Grob, "Dimensional models of core affect: a quantitative comparison by means of structural equation modeling," *European Journal of Personality,* vol. 14, no. 4, pp. 325-345, 2000.

[20] M. Bradley, And P. Lang, "Measuring Emotion - The Self-Assessment Mannequin And The Semantic Differential," *Journal of Behavior Therapy and Experimental Psychiatry,* vol. 25, no. 1, pp. 49-59, MAR 1994, 1994.

[21] P. Ekman, W. Friesen, M. Osullivan, A. Chan, I. Diacoyannitarlatzis, K. Heider, R. Krause, W. Lecompte, T. Pitcairn, P. Riccibitti, K. Scherer, M. Tomita, And A. Tzavaras, "Universals And Cultural-Differences In The Judgments Of Facial Expressions Of Emotion," *Journal Of Personality And Social Psychology,* Vol. 53, No. 4, Pp. 712-717, Oct 1987, 1987.

[22] P. Ekman, and W. V. Friesen, "Constants Across Cultures in the Face and Emotion," *Journal of Personality and Social Psychology,* vol. 17, no. 2, pp. 124-129., 1971.

[23] J. Russell, "Culture And The Categorization Of Emotions," *Psychological Bulletin,* Vol. 110, No. 3, Pp. 426-450, Nov 1991, 1991.

[24] P. Ekman, "Are There Basic Emotions," *Psychological Review,* vol. 99, no. 3, pp. 550-553, Jul 1992, 1992.

[25] R. Levenson, "Basic Emotion Questions," *Emotion Review,* vol. 3, no. 4, pp. 379-386, Oct 2011, 2011.

[26] A. Al-Nafjan, M. Hosny, Y. Al-Ohali, and A. Al-Wabil, "Review and Classification of Emotion Recognition Based on EEG Brain-Computer Interface System Research: A Systematic Review," *Applied Sciences-Basel,* vol. 7, no. 12, Dec 2017, 2017.

[27] M. Bradley, S. Hamby, A. Low, and P. Lang, "Brain potentials in perception: Picture complexity and emotional arousal," *Psychophysiology,* vol. 44, no. 3, pp. 364-373, May 2007, 2007.

[28] J. Olofsson, S. Nordin, H. Sequeira, and J. Polich, "Affective picture processing: An integrative review of ERP findings," *Biological Psychology,* vol. 77, no. 3, pp. 247-265, Mar 2008, 2008.

[29] A. Gabrielsson, "Emotions in strong experiences with music.," *Music and emotion: Theory and research*, P. Juslin, Sloboda, J.A., ed., pp. 431-449, Oxford, UK: Oxford University Press, 2001.

[30] L. Balkwill, and W. Thompson, "A cross-cultural investigation of the perception of emotion in music: Psychophysical and cultural cues," *Music Perception,* vol. 17, no. 1, pp. 43-64, Fal 1999, 1999.

[31] I. Molnar-Szakacs, and K. Overy, "Music and mirror neurons: from motion to 'e'motion," *Social Cognitive and Affective Neuroscience,* vol. 1, no. 3, pp. 235-241, Dec 2006, 2006.

[32] D. Brown, and J. Cavanagh, "The sound and the fury: Late positive potential is sensitive to sound affect," *Psychophysiology,* vol. 54, no. 12, pp. 1812-1825, Dec 2017, 2017.

[33] L. Thomas, and K. LaBar, "Emotional arousal enhances word repetition priming," *Cognition & Emotion,* vol. 19, no. 7, pp. 1027-1047, Nov 2005, 2005.

[34] M. Zhang, Y. Ge, C. Kang, T. Guo, and D. Peng, "ERP evidence for the contribution of meaning complexity underlying emotional word processing,"

Journal of Neurolinguistics, vol. 45, pp. 110-118, Feb 2018, 2018.

[35] J. Kline, G. Blackhart, K. Woodward, S. Williams, and G. Schwartz, "Anterior electroencephalographic asymmetry changes in elderly women in response to a pleasant and an unpleasant odor," *Biological Psychology,* vol. 52, no. 3, pp. 241-250, Apr 2000, 2000.

[36] E. Kroupi, J. Vesin, and T. Ebrahimi, "Subject-Independent Odor Pleasantness Classification Using Brain and Peripheral Signals," *IEEE Transactions on Affective Computing,* vol. 7, no. 4, pp. 422-434, Oct-Dec 2016, 2016.

[37] A. Novosel, N. Lackner, H. Unterrainer, M. Dunitz-Scheer, P. Scheer, S. Wallner-Liebmann, and C. Neuper, "Motivational processing of food cues in anorexia nervosa: a pilot study," *Eating and Weight Disorders-Studies on Anorexia Bulimia and Obesity,* vol. 19, no. 2, pp. 169-175, Jun 2014, 2014.

[38] U. o. Surrey. "Surrey Audio-Visual Expressed Emotion (SAVEE) database," http://kahlan.eps.surrey.ac.uk/savee/.

[39] P. J. Lang, M. M. Bradley, and B. N. Cuthbert, *International affective picture system (IAPS): Affective ratings of pictures and instruction manual. Technical Report A-8.*, University ofFlorida, Gainesville, FL., 2008.

[40] M. M. Bradley, and P. J. Lang, *The International Affective Digitized Sounds (2nd Edition; IADS-2): Affective ratings of sounds and instruction manual. Technical report B-3.*, University of Florida, Gainesville, Fl., 2007.

[41] M. M. Bradley, and P. J. Lang, *Affective Norms for English Words (ANEW): Instruction manual and affective ratings. Technical Report C-3.*, UF Center for the Study of Emotion and Attention. Gainesville, FL., 2017.

[42] M. M. Bradley, and P. J. Lang, *Affective Norms for English Text (ANET): Affective ratings of text and instruction manual. (Tech. Rep. No. D-1).* University of Florida, Gainesville, FL., 2007.

[43] S. Livingstone, and F. Russo, "The Ryerson Audio-Visual Database of Emotional Speech and Song (RAVDESS): A dynamic, multimodal set of facial and vocal expressions in North American English," *Plos One,* vol. 13, no. 5, May 16 2018, 2018.

[44] S. Paquette, I. Peretz, and B. Pascal, "Can We Dissociate The Musical Emotional Pathway From The Vocal One?," *Journal of Cognitive Neuroscience*, pp. 214-214, 2013, 2013.

[45] G. Pfurtscheller, And A. Aranibar, "Event-Related Cortical Desynchronization Detected By Power Measurements Of Scalp EEG," *Electroencephalography and Clinical Neurophysiology,* vol. 42, no. 6, pp. 817-826, 1977, 1977.

[46] G. Pfurtscheller, and F. da Silva, "Event-related EEG/MEG synchronization and desynchronization: basic principles," *Clinical Neurophysiology,* vol. 110, no. 11, pp. 1842-1857, Nov 1999, 1999.

[47] S. van den Broek, F. Reinders, M. Donderwinkel, and M. Peters, "Volume conduction effects in EEG and MEG," *Electroencephalography and Clinical Neurophysiology,* vol. 106, no. 6, pp. 522-534, JUN 1998, 1998.

[48] R. Pascualmarqui, C. Michel, And D. Lehmann, "Low-Resolution Electromagnetic Tomography - A New Method For Localizing Electrical-Activity In The Brain," *International Journal of Psychophysiology,* vol. 18, no. 1, pp. 49-65, Oct 1994, 1994.

[49] R. Khemakhem, W. Zouch, A. Ben Hamida, A. Taleb-Ahmed, and I. Feki, "EEG Source Localization Using the

Inverse Problem Methods," *International Journal of Computer Science and Network Security,* vol. 9, no. 4, pp. 408-415, Apr 30 2009, 2009.

[50] C. Michel, M. Murray, G. Lantz, S. Gonzalez, L. Spinelli, and R. de Peralta, "EEG source imaging," *Clinical Neurophysiology,* vol. 115, no. 10, pp. 2195-2222, Oct 2004, 2004.

[51] A. Neuro. "Electrodes Layout," 06/06/2019; https://www.ant-neuro.com/products/waveguard/electrode-layouts.

[52] A. Cohen, D. Fair, N. Dosenbach, F. Miezin, D. Dierker, D. Van Essen, B. Schlaggar, and S. Petersen, "Defining functional areas in individual human brains using resting functional connectivity MRI," *Neuroimage,* vol. 41, no. 1, pp. 45-57, May 15 2008, 2008.

[53] M. Lindquist, "The Statistical Analysis of fMRI Data," *Statistical Science,* vol. 23, no. 4, pp. 439-464, Nov 2008, 2008.

[54] C. Gerloff, W. Grodd, E. Altenmuller, R. Kolb, T. Naegele, U. Klose, K. Voigt, and J. Dichgans, "Coregistration of EEG and fMRI in a simple motor task," *Human Brain Mapping,* vol. 4, no. 3, pp. 199-209, 1996, 1996.

[55] R. Labounek, D. Bridwell, R. Marecek, M. Lamos, M. Mikl, P. Bednarik, J. Bastinec, T. Slavicek, P. Hlustik, M. Brazdil, and J. Jan, "EEG spatiospectral patterns and their link to fMRI BOLD signal via variable hemodynamic response functions," *Journal of Neuroscience Methods,* vol. 318, pp. 34-46, Apr 15 2019, 2019.

[56] V. Salmela, E. Salo, J. Salmi, and K. Alho, "Spatiotemporal Dynamics of Attention Networks Revealed by Representational Similarity Analysis of EEG and fMRI," *Cerebral Cortex,* vol. 28, no. 2, pp. 549-560, FEB 2018, 2018.

[57] R. Ahmad, A. Malik, N. Kamel, F. Reza, H. Amin, and M. Hussain, "Visual brain activity patterns classification with simultaneous EEG-fMRI: A multimodal approach," *Technology and Health Care,* vol. 25, no. 3, pp. 471-485, 2017, 2017.

[58] Q. Guo, T. Zhou, W. Li, L. Dong, S. Wang, and L. Zou, "Single-trial EEG-informed fMRI analysis of emotional decision problems in hot executive function," *Brain and Behavior,* vol. 7, no. 7, Jul 2017, 2017.

[59] J. Bodurka, "Amygdala Emotional Regulation Training With Real-Time fMRI Neurofeedback and Concurrent EEG Recordings," *Biological Psychiatry,* vol. 83, no. 9, pp. S58-S58, May 1 2018, 2018.

[60] A. Babayan, M. Erbey, D. Kumral, J. Reinelt, A. Reiter, J. Roebbig, H. Schaare, M. Uhlig, A. Anwander, P. Bazin, A. Horstmann, L. Lampe, V. Nikulin, H. Okon-Singer, S. Preusser, A. Pampel, C. Rohr, J. Sacher, A. Thoene-Otto, S. Trapp, T. Nierhaus, D. Altmann, K. Arelin, M. Bloechl, E. Bongartz, P. Breig, E. Cesnaite, S. Chen, R. Cozatl, S. Czerwonatis, G. Dambrauskaite, M. Dreyer, J. Enders, M. Engelhardt, M. Fischer, N. Forschack, J. Golchert, L. Golz, C. Guran, S. Hedrich, N. Hentschel, D. Hoffmann, J. Huntenburg, R. Jost, A. Kosatschek, S. Kunzendorf, H. Lammers, M. Lauckner, K. Mahjoory, A. Kanaan, N. Mendes, R. Menger, E. Morino, K. Naethe, J. Neubauer, H. Noyan, S. Oligschlaeger, P. Panczyszyn-Trzewik, D. Poehlchen, N. Putzke, S. Roski, M. Schaller, A. Schieferbein, B. Schlaak, R. Schmidt, K. Gorgolewski, H. Schmidt, A. Schrimpf, S. Stasch, M. Voss, A. Wiedemann, D. Margulies, M. Gaebler, and A. Villringer, "A mind-brain-body dataset of MRI, EEG, cognition, emotion, and peripheral physiology in young and old adults," *Scientific Data,* vol. 6, Feb 12 2019, 2019.

[61] M. Schrooten, R. Vandenberghe, R. Peeters, and P. Dupont, "Quantitative

Analyses Help in Choosing Between Simultaneous vs. Separate EEG and fMRI," *Frontiers in Neuroscience,* vol. 12, Jan 10 2019, 2019.

[62] R. Abreu, A. Leal, and P. Figueiredo, "EEG-Informed fMRI: A Review of Data Analysis Methods," *Frontiers in Human Neuroscience,* vol. 12, Feb 6 2018, 2018.

[63] K. Friston, J. Ashburner, S. Kiebel, T. Nichols, and W. Penny, "Statistical Parametric Mapping: The Analysis of Functional Brain Images," *Statistical Parametric Mapping: the Analysis of Functional Brain Images*, pp. 1-680, 2007, 2007.

[64] iMotions, *EEG (Eectroencephalography): The Complete Pocket Guide*, 2017.

[65] S. Koelstra, C. Muhl, M. Soleymani, J. Lee, A. Yazdani, T. Ebrahimi, T. Pun, A. Nijholt, and I. Patras, "DEAP: A Database for Emotion Analysis Using Physiological Signals," *IEEE Transactions on Affective Computing,* vol. 3, no. 1, pp. 18-31, Jan-Mar 2012, 2012.

[66] J. Coan, and J. Allen, "Frontal EEG asymmetry as a moderator and mediator of emotion," *Biological Psychology,* vol. 67, no. 1-2, pp. 7-49, OCT 2004, 2004.

[67] G. Hajcak, A. MacNamara, and D. Olvet, "Event-Related Potentials, Emotion, and Emotion Regulation: An Integrative Review," *Developmental Neuropsychology,* vol. 35, no. 2, pp. 129-155, 2010, 2010.

[68] L. Carretie, J. Hinojosa, M. Martin-Loeches, F. Mercado, and M. Tapia, "Automatic attention to emotional stimuli: Neural correlates," *Human Brain Mapping,* vol. 22, no. 4, pp. 290-299, AUG 2004, 2004.

[69] H. Schupp, M. Junghofer, A. Weike, and A. Hamm, "Emotional facilitation of sensory processing in the visual cortex," *Psychological Science,* vol. 14, no. 1, pp. 7-13, Jan 2003, 2003.

[70] H. Schupp, B. Cuthbert, M. Bradley, C. Hillman, A. Hamm, and P. Lang, "Brain processes in emotional perception: Motivated attention," *Cognition & Emotion,* vol. 18, no. 5, pp. 593-611, AUG 2004, 2004.

[71] H. Schupp, A. Ohman, M. Junghofer, A. Weike, J. Stockburger, and A. Hamm, "The facilitated processing of threatening faces: An ERP analysis," *Emotion,* vol. 4, no. 2, pp. 189-200, Jun 2004, 2004.

[72] I. Franken, L. Gootjes, and J. van Strien, "Automatic processing of emotional words during an emotional Stroop task," *Neuroreport,* vol. 20, no. 8, pp. 776-781, May 27 2009, 2009.

[73] R. Johnson, "For Distinguished Early Career Contribution To Psychophysiology - Award Address, 1985 - A Triarchic Model Of P300 Amplitude," *Psychophysiology,* vol. 23, no. 4, pp. 367-384, Jul 1986, 1986.

[74] A. Mini, D. Palomba, A. Angrilli, and S. Bravi, "Emotional information processing and visual evoked brain potentials," *Perceptual and Motor Skills,* vol. 83, no. 1, pp. 143-152, Aug 1996, 1996.

[75] J. Radilova, "The Late Positive Component Of Visual Evoked-Response Sensitive To Emotional Factors," *Activitas Nervosa Superior*, pp. 334-337, 1982, 1982.

[76] D. Palomba, A. Angrilli, and A. Mini, "Visual evoked potentials, heart rate responses and memory to emotional pictorial stimuli," *International Journal of Psychophysiology,* vol. 27, no. 1, pp. 55-67, Jul 1997, 1997.

[77] B. Cuthbert, M. Bradley, and P. Lang, "Probing picture

perception: Activation and emotion," *Psychophysiology,* vol. 33, no. 2, pp. 103-111, Mar 1996, 1996.

[78] T. Suo, L. Liu, C. Chen, and E. Zhang, "The Functional Role of Individual-Alpha Based Frontal Asymmetry in the Evaluation of Emotional Pictures: Evidence from Event-Related Potentials," *Frontiers in Psychiatry,* vol. 8, Sep 27 2017, 2017.

[79] M. Codispoti, V. Ferrari, and M. Bradley, "Repetition and event-related potentials: Distinguishing early and late processes in affective picture perception," *Journal of Cognitive Neuroscience,* vol. 19, no. 4, pp. 577-586, Apr 2007, 2007.

[80] J. Olofsson, and J. Polich, "Affective visual event-related potentials: Arousal, repetition, and time-on-task," *Biological Psychology,* vol. 75, no. 1, pp. 101-108, Apr 2007, 2007.

[81] M. Bradley, "Natural selective attention: Orienting and emotion," *Psychophysiology,* vol. 46, no. 1, pp. 1-11, Jan 2009, 2009.

[82] P. Lang, M. Bradley, J. Fitzsimmons, B. Cuthbert, J. Scott, B. Moulder, and V. Nangia, "Emotional arousal and activation of the visual cortex: An fMRI analysis," *Psychophysiology,* vol. 35, no. 2, pp. 199-210, Mar 1998, 1998.

[83] S. Moon, and J. Lee, "Implicit Analysis of Perceptual Multimedia Experience Based on Physiological Response: A Review," *IEEE Transactions on Multimedia,* vol. 19, no. 2, pp. 340-353, Feb 2017, 2017.

[84] L. Gianotti, *P. Faber*, M. Schuler, R. Pascual-Marqui, K. Kochi, and D. Lehmann, "First valence, then arousal: The temporal dynamics of brain electric activity evoked by emotional stimuli," *Brain Topography,* vol. 20, no. 3, pp. 143-156, Mar 2008, 2008.

[85] E. Bernat, S. Bunce, and H. Shevrin, "Event-related brain potentials differentiate positive and negative mood adjectives during both supraliminal and subliminal visual processing," *International Journal of Psychophysiology,* vol. 42, no. 1, pp. 11-34, Aug 2001, 2001.

[86] R. Roschmann, And W. Wittling, "Topographic Brain Mapping Of Emotion-Related Hemisphere Asymmetries," *International Journal of Neuroscience,* vol. 63, no. 1-2, pp. 5-16, 1992, 1992.

[87] M. Kim, M. Kim, E. Oh, and S. Kim, "A Review on the Computational Methods for Emotional State Estimation from the Human EEG," *Computational and Mathematical Methods in Medicine*, 2013, 2013.

[88] C. Di Dio, E. Macaluso, and G. Rizzolatti, "The Golden Beauty: Brain Response to Classical and Renaissance Sculptures," *Plos One,* vol. 2, no. 11, Nov 21 2007, 2007.

[89] E. Phelps, and J. LeDoux, "Contributions of the amygdala to emotion processing: From animal models to human behavior," *Neuron,* vol. 48, no. 2, pp. 175-187, OCT 20 2005, 2005.

[90] B. Knutson, C. Adams, G. Fong, and D. Hommer, "Anticipation of increasing monetary reward selectively recruits nucleus accumbens," *Journal of Neuroscience,* vol. 21, no. 16, pp. art. no.-RC159, Aug 15 2001, 2001.

[91] H. Breiter, I. Aharon, D. Kahneman, *A. dale*, and P. Shizgal, "Functional imaging of neural responses to expectancy and experience of monetary gains and losses," *Neuron,* vol. 30, no. 2, pp. 619-639, May 2001, 2001.

[92] V. Menon, and D. Levitin, "The rewards of music listening: Response and physiological connectivity of the

mesolimbic system," *Neuroimage,* vol. 28, no. 1, pp. 175-184, Oct 15 2005, 2005.

[93] A. Blood, and R. Zatorre, "Intensely pleasurable responses to music correlate with activity in brain regions implicated in reward and emotion," *Proceedings of the National Academy of Sciences of the United States of America,* vol. 98, no. 20, pp. 11818-11823, Sep 25 2001, 2001.

[94] G. Bush, P. Luu, and M. Posner, "Cognitive and emotional influences in anterior cingulate cortex," *Trends in Cognitive Sciences,* vol. 4, no. 6, pp. 215-222, Jun 2000, 2000.

[95] A. Bechara, H. Damasio, and A. Damasio, "Emotion, decision making and the orbitofrontal cortex," *Cerebral Cortex,* vol. 10, no. 3, pp. 295-307, Mar 2000, 2000.

[96] S. Koelsch, T. Fritz, K. Schulze, D. Alsop, and G. Schlaug, "Adults and children processing music: An fMR1 study," *Neuroimage,* vol. 25, no. 4, pp. 1068-1076, May 1 2005, 2005.

[97] S. Koelsch, T. Fritz, D. Von Cramon, K. Muller, and A. Friederici, "Investigating emotion with music: An fMRI study," *Human Brain Mapping,* vol. 27, no. 3, pp. 239-250, Mar 2006, 2006.

[98] H. Kawabata, and S. Zeki, "Neural correlates of beauty," *Journal of Neurophysiology,* vol. 91, no. 4, pp. 1699-1705, Apr 2004, 2004.

[99] D. Cinzia, and G. Vittorio, "Neuroaesthetics: a review," *Current Opinion in Neurobiology,* vol. 19, no. 6, pp. 682-687, Dec 2009, 2009.

[100] L. Schmidt, and L. Trainor, "Frontal brain electrical activity (EEG) distinguishes valence and intensity of musical emotions," *Cognition & Emotion,* vol. 15, no. 4, pp. 487-500, Jul 2001, 2001.

[101] L. Carr, M. Iacoboni, M. Dubeau, J. Mazziotta, and G. Lenzi, "Neural mechanisms of empathy in humans: A relay from neural systems for imitation to limbic areas," *Proceedings of the National Academy of Sciences of the United States of America,* vol. 100, no. 9, pp. 5497-5502, Apr 29 2003, 2003.

[102] A. Craig, "How do you feel? Interoception: the sense of the physiological condition of the body," *Nature Reviews Neuroscience,* vol. 3, no. 8, pp. 655-666, Aug 2002, 2002.

[103] A. Craig, "Human feelings: why are some more aware than others?," *Trends in Cognitive Sciences,* vol. 8, no. 6, pp. 239-241, Jun 2004, 2004.

[104] H. Critchley, S. Wiens, P. Rotshtein, A. Ohman, and R. Dolan, "Neural systems supporting interoceptive awareness," *Nature Neuroscience,* vol. 7, no. 2, pp. 189-195, Feb 2004, 2004.

[105] Y. Lin, Y. Yang, and T. Jung, "Fusion of electroencephalographic dynamics and musical contents for estimating emotional responses in music listening," *Frontiers in Neuroscience,* vol. 8, May 1 2014, 2014.

[106] M. Wyczesany, S. Grzybowski, R. Barry, J. Kaiser, A. Coenen, and A. Potoczek, "Covariation of EEG Synchronization and Emotional State as Modified by Anxiolytics," *Journal of Clinical Neurophysiology,* vol. 28, no. 3, pp. 289-296, Jun 2011, 2011.

[107] V. Miskovic, and L. Schmidt, "Cross-regional cortical synchronization during affective image viewing," *Brain Research,* vol. 1362, pp. 102-111, Nov 29 2010, 2010.

[108] *N. martini*, D. Menicucci, L. Sebastiani, R. Bedini, A. Pingitore, N. Vanello, M. Milanesi, L. Landini, and A. Gemignani, "The dynamics of EEG gamma responses to unpleasant visual

stimuli: From local activity to functional connectivity," *Neuroimage,* vol. 60, no. 2, pp. 922-932, Apr 2 2012, 2012.

[109] C. Han, J. Lee, J. Lim, Y. Kim, and C. Im, "Global Electroencephalography Synchronization as a New Indicator for Tracking Emotional Changes of a Group of Individuals during Video Watching," *Frontiers in Human Neuroscience,* vol. 11, Dec 1 2017, 2017.

[110] L. Fogassi, and G. Luppino, "Motor functions of the parietal lobe," *Current Opinion in Neurobiology,* vol. 15, no. 6, pp. 626-631, DEC 2005, 2005.

[111] T. Jacobsen, R. Schubotz, L. Hofel, and D. Von Cramon, "Brain correlates of aesthetic judgment of beauty," *Neuroimage,* vol. 29, no. 1, pp. 276-285, Jan 1 2006, 2006.

[112] D. Jackson, C. Mueller, I. Dolski, K. Dalton, J. Nitschke, H. Urry, M. Rosenkranz, C. Ryff, B. Singer, and R. Davidson, "Now you feel it, now you don't: Frontal brain electrical asymmetry and individual differences in emotion regulation," *Psychological Science,* vol. 14, no. 6, pp. 612-617, Nov 2003, 2003.

[113] S. Edwards, D. Everhart, H. Demaree, and D. Harrison, "Sex-related electroencephalographic differences observed during positive and negative affective verbal learning," *Psychophysiology,* vol. 43, pp. S36-S36, 2006, 2006.

[114] J. Hardee, L. Cope, E. Munier, R. Welsh, R. Zucker, and M. Heitzeg, "Sex differences in the development of emotion circuitry in adolescents at risk for substance abuse: a longitudinal fMRI study," *Social Cognitive and Affective Neuroscience,* vol. 12, no. 6, pp. 965-975, Jun 2017, 2017.

[115] C. Cela-Conde, F. Ayala, E. Munar, F. Maestu, M. Nadal, M. Capo, D. del Rio, J. Lopez-Ibor, T. Ortiz, C. Mirasso, and G. Marty, "Sex-related similarities and differences in the neural correlates of beauty," *Proceedings of the National Academy of Sciences of the United States of America,* vol. 106, no. 10, pp. 3847-3852, Mar 10 2009, 2009.

Chapter 2

Modeling of the Flexible Needle Insertion into the Human Liver

Veturia Chiroiu, Ligia Munteanu, Cristian Rugină and Nicoleta Nedelcu

Abstract

The insertion of the needle is difficult because the deformation and displacement of the organs are the key elements in the surgical act. Liver and tumor modeling are essential in the development of the needle insertion model. The role of the needle is to deliver into the tumor an active chemotherapeutic agent. We describe in this chapter the deformation of the needle during its insertion into the human liver in the context of surgery simulation of the high- robotic-assisted intraoperative treatment of liver tumors based on the integrated imaging-molecular diagnosis. The needle is a bee barbed type modeled as a flexible thread within the framework of the Cosserat (micropolar) elasticity theory.

Keywords: bee needle, human liver, Cosserat elasticity theory

1. Introduction

The flexible bee needles are useful tools to transport drugs into the liver tumors [1, 2]. The insertion trajectory of the needle must avoid the ribs, blood vessels, and other organs to protect the liver [3–6] (**Figure 1a**). The bee needle assures reduced insertion forces and small tissue deformations because of the tip deflections. The furthermost current publications on the surgical needle navigation into the liver can be demonstrated in [7–9]. The bee needle is shown in **Figure 1b**. The front angle has 157 deg., the back angle, 110 deg., the height is 0.5 mm, and the tip thickness 0.15 mm.

A number of scientific researches have been carried out on the collision free trajectory of the needle to the target. The surgical event requires experience in imaging the tumor location based on the liver structure and the microstructural interaction between the needle and the liver. Several studies have revealed that the needle flexibility is essential to achieve a good precision in the handling.

The strain and stress fields and the topological changes of the liver are not to be neglected during the needle navigation towards the tumor [10–13]. Details of the forces during needle insertion into the liver are find in [14], the real time collision detection for virtual surgery in [15] and the minimal hierarchical collision detection in [16]. Optimization is required to modify the needle trajectory in order to protect the liver [17, 18], to manage the tumor risk [19], and to change the robot architecture [20–22]. The inverse sonification problem for capturing hardly detectable details in a medical image is treated in [23], and the control in [24–27]. Microscopic investigation of the human liver offers details on its microanatomy with emphases

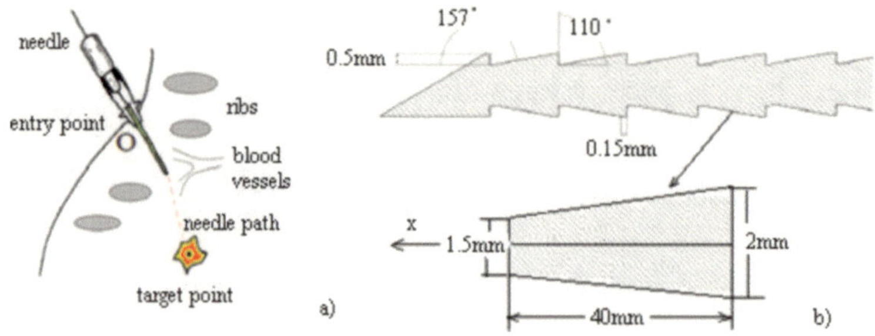

Figure 1.
a) Trajectory towards the liver tumor; b) honeybee barbed needle [1, 2].

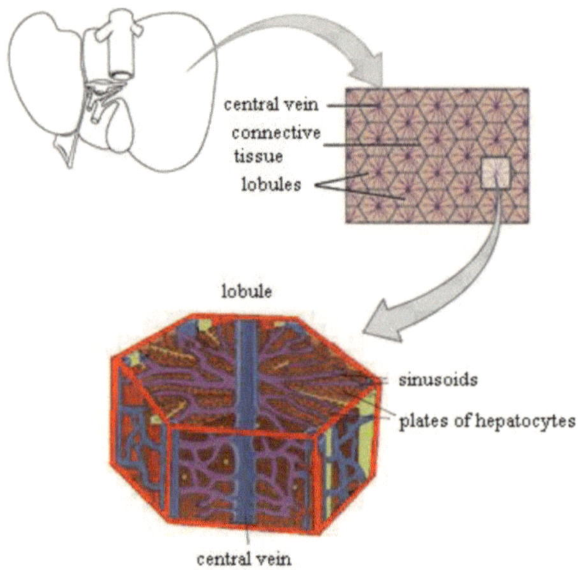

Figure 2.
Hepatic lobule - basic unit of the liver.

to the granular, fibrillar components and irregular solid–fluid interfaces [28–30]. The basic unit of the liver is the hepatic lobule which is a hexagonal element with comprised the portal triad -portal vein, hepatic artery and the bile duct [31, 32]. Lobuli form two layers membranes with internal space of 100A and the cellular elements with twisted, spiraling fibers braided into the helical and screw-shaped gaps (pores) of 40–100 μm in size (**Figure 2**) [33–36].

In this chapter we try to answer a few questions such as how is the deformation of the needle and how the free-collision trajectories are determined.

2. Deformation of the needle

The needle is a bee barbed needle and it is modeled as a flexible thread within the framework of the Cosserat (micropolar) elasticity theory [37–42]. The Cosserat elasticity is applied to describe the interaction between the needle and the human liver. Let us consider a serial surgical robot composed of a revolute joint and a flexible needle. A Lagrange frame (X, Y, Z) of base vectors (e_1, e_2, e_3) and origin O in the entry point of the skin is attached to the robot (**Figure 3**). The Euler frame $K(x, y, z)$ with origin in the joint and the base vectors (d_1, d_2, d_3) is attached to the

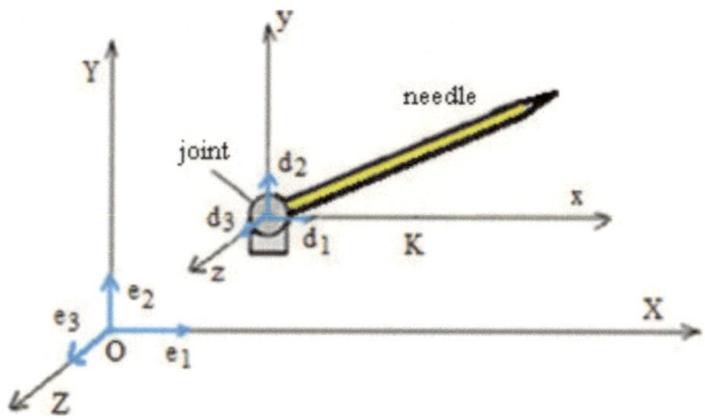

Figure 3.
Lagrange coordinate system OXYZ and the Euler coordinate system oxyz attached to the needle.

needle. The angle between the flexible arm and axis x is θ. Bending and torsion of the needle are described by the strain functions (u_1, u_2, u_3). The robot has f degrees of freedom $f = f_r + f_e$, where $f_r = 1$ is the generalized coordinate of the rigid system and $f_e = 3$ are the degrees of freedom of the flexible needle [43, 44].

The Euler axes are oriented with respect to the Lagrange axes by Euler angles υ, ψ and φ [43].

$$\begin{aligned} d_1 &= (-\sin\psi\sin\varphi + \cos\psi\cos\varphi\cos\upsilon)e_1 + \\ &\quad +(\cos\psi\sin\varphi + \sin\psi\cos\varphi\cos\upsilon)e_2 - \sin\upsilon\cos\varphi e_3, \\ d_2 &= (-\sin\psi\cos\varphi - \cos\psi\sin\varphi\cos\upsilon)e_1 + \\ &\quad +(\cos\psi\cos\varphi - \sin\psi\sin\varphi\cos\upsilon)e_2 + \sin\upsilon\sin\varphi e_3, \\ d_3 &= \sin\upsilon\cos\psi e_1 + \sin\upsilon\sin\psi e_2 + \cos\upsilon\, e_3. \end{aligned} \tag{1}$$

The functions (u_1, u_2, u_3) measure the bending and torsion of the needle as

$$\begin{aligned} u_1 &= \upsilon'\sin\varphi - \psi'\sin\upsilon\cos\varphi, \\ u_2 &= \upsilon'\cos\varphi + \psi'\sin\upsilon\sin\varphi, \\ u_3 &= \varphi' + \psi'\cos\upsilon, \end{aligned} \tag{2}$$

where $(')$ means the partial differentiation with respect to s which is the coordinate along the central line of the needle. The functions u_1 and u_2 describe the bending of the needle, and the function u_3 the torsion of the needle. In addition, u_1 and u_2 are components of the curvature κ of the central line corresponding to the planes (yz) and (xz)

$$\kappa^2 = u_1^2 + u_2^2 = \upsilon'^2 + \psi'^2\sin^2\upsilon. \tag{3}$$

The function u_3 measures the torsion τ of the needle

$$u_3 = \tau = \varphi' + \psi'\cos\upsilon. \tag{4}$$

So, the needle is rigid along the tangential direction and the total length of the needle l is invariant, the ends being fixed by the force $F = -f$ with $f = (f_1, f_2, f_3)$. This force describes the contact between the needle and the tissue $f = p_c n = p_c g'$, where g is a gap function with respect to s.

The link between the position vector $r = (x, y, z)$ and unit tangential vector d_3 is $r = \int_0^s d_3 \, ds$, or

$$x(s) = \int_0^s \cos\psi \sin\upsilon \, ds, y(s) = \int_0^s \sin\psi \sin\upsilon \, ds, z(s) = \int_0^s \cos\upsilon \, ds. \tag{5}$$

We introduce the inertia of the needle characterized by

$$(\rho_0 A_0)(s), (\rho_0 I_1)(s), (\rho_0 I_2(s)), \tag{6}$$

where ρ_0 is the mass density per unit volume, A_0 the area of the cross section, I_1, I_2 are geometrical moments of inertia around the axis, which is perpendicular to the central axis and respectively around the central axis.

The equations which describe the deformation are

$$-\rho\ddot{r} - \lambda' = 0, \tag{7}$$

$$\begin{aligned} & k_1\left(\dot{\psi}^2 \sin\upsilon\cos\upsilon - \ddot{\upsilon}\right) - k_2(\dot{\varphi} + \dot{\psi}\cos\upsilon)\,\dot{\psi}\sin\upsilon - \\ & -A\left(\psi'^2 \sin\upsilon\cos\upsilon - \upsilon''\right) + C(\varphi' + \psi'\cos\upsilon)\psi'\sin\upsilon - \\ & -\lambda_1\cos\upsilon\cos\psi - \lambda_2\cos\upsilon\sin\psi + \lambda_3\sin\upsilon = 0, \end{aligned} \tag{8}$$

$$\begin{aligned} & -\frac{\partial}{\partial t}\{k_1\dot{\psi}\sin^2\upsilon + k_2(\dot{\varphi} + \dot{\psi}\cos\upsilon)\cos\upsilon\} + \\ & +\frac{\partial}{\partial s}\left\{A\psi'^2\sin^2\upsilon + C(\varphi' + \psi'\cos\upsilon)\cos\upsilon\right\} + \\ & +\lambda_1\sin\upsilon\sin\psi - \lambda_2\sin\upsilon\cos\psi = 0, \end{aligned} \tag{9}$$

$$-k_2\frac{\partial}{\partial t}(\dot{\varphi} + \dot{\psi}\cos\upsilon) + C\frac{\partial}{\partial s}(\varphi' + \psi'\cos\upsilon) = 0. \tag{10}$$

where A and C are the bending stiffness and respectively the torsional stiffness of the needle, related to the Lame constants λ, μ by $A = \frac{1}{4}\pi a^4 E, C = \frac{1}{2}\pi a^4 \mu, A = \frac{1}{4}\pi a^4 E, C = \frac{1}{2}\pi a^4 \mu$, where $E = \frac{\mu(3\lambda+2\mu)}{\lambda+\mu}$ is the Young's elastic modulus, and a is the radius of the cross section of the needle, and

$$\rho = A_0\rho_0 = \pi a^2\rho_0, k_1 = I_1\rho_0 = \frac{\pi a^4}{4}\rho_0, k_2 = I_2\rho_0 = \frac{\pi a^4}{2}\rho_0. \tag{11}$$

The Eqs. (7–11) are solved by using the cnoidal method [43].

In short, this method is reducible to a generalization of the Fourier series with the cnoidal functions as the fundamental basis function. This is because the cnoidal functions are much richer than the trigonometric or hyperbolic functions, that is, the modulus m of the cnoidal function, $0 \le m \le 1$, can be varied to obtain a sine or cosine function ($m \cong 0$), a Stokes function ($m \cong 0.5$) or a solitonic function, sech or tanh.

To understand the cnoidal method, consider now a nonlinear system of equations that govern the motion of a dynamical system

$$\frac{d\theta_i}{dt} = F_i(\theta_1, \theta_2, \ldots, \theta_n), i = 1, \ldots, n, n \ge 3, \tag{12}$$

with $x \in \mathrm{R}^n$, $t \in [0, T]$, $T \in R$, where F may be of the form

$$F_i = \sum_{p=1}^{n} a_{ip}\theta_p + \sum_{p,q=1}^{n} b_{ipq}\theta_p\theta_q + \sum_{p,q,r=1}^{n} c_{ipqr}\theta_p\theta_q\theta_r + \\ + \sum_{p,q,r,l=1}^{n} d_{ipqrl}\theta_p\theta_q\theta_r\theta_l + \sum_{p,q,r,l,m=1}^{n} e_{ipqrlm}\theta_p\theta_q\theta_r\theta_l\theta_m + \dots, \tag{13}$$

where $i = 1, 2, \dots, n$, and $a, b, c \dots$ constants.
This system of equations can be reduced to Weierstrass equations of the type

$$\dot{\theta}_2 = P_n(\theta), \tag{14}$$

We introduce the function transformation

$$\theta = 2\frac{\mathrm{d}^2}{\mathrm{d}t} \log \Theta_n(t), \tag{15}$$

where the theta function $\Theta_n(t)$ are defined as

$$\begin{gathered} \Theta_1 = 1 + \exp(\mathrm{i}\omega_1 t + B_{11}), \\ \Theta_2 = 1 + \exp(\mathrm{i}\omega_1 t + B_{11}) + \exp(\mathrm{i}\omega_2 t + B_{22}) + \exp(\omega_1 + \omega_2 + B_{12}), \\ \Theta_3 = 1 + \exp(\mathrm{i}\omega_1 t + B_{11}) + \exp(\mathrm{i}\omega_2 t + B_{22}) + \\ + \exp(\mathrm{i}\omega_3 t + B_{33}) + \exp(\omega_1 + \omega_2 + B_{12}) + \\ + \exp(\omega_1 + \omega_3 + B_{13}) + \exp(\omega_2 + \omega_3 + B_{23}) + \\ + \exp(\omega_1 + \omega_2 + \omega_3 + B_{12} + B_{13} + B_{23}), \end{gathered} \tag{16}$$

and

$$\Theta_n = \sum_{M \in (-\infty, \infty)} \exp\left(\mathrm{i}\sum_{i=1}^{n} M_i\omega_i t + \frac{1}{2}\sum_{i<j}^{n} B_{ij}M_iM_j\right), \tag{17}$$

$$\exp B_{ij} = \left(\frac{\omega_i - \omega_j}{\omega_i + \omega_j}\right)^2, \ \exp B_{ii} = \omega_i^2. \tag{18}$$

Further, we write the solution (15) under the form

$$\theta(t) = 2\frac{\partial^2}{\partial t^2} \log \Theta_n(\eta) = \theta_{lin}(\eta) + \theta_{int}(\eta), \tag{19}$$

for $\eta = -\omega t + \phi$. The first term θ_{lin} represents a linear superposition of cnoidal waves. Indeed, after a little manipulation and algebraic calculus, obtain

$$\theta_{lin} = \sum_{l=1}^{n} \alpha_l \left[\frac{2\pi}{K_l\sqrt{m_l}} \sum_{k=0}^{\infty} \left[\frac{q_l^{k+1/2}}{1 + q_l^{2k+1}} \cos(2k+1)\frac{\pi\omega_l t}{2K_l}\right]^2\right]. \tag{20}$$

In (20) we recognize the expression [43].

$$\theta_{lin} = \sum_{l=1}^{n} \alpha_l \,\mathrm{cn}^2[\omega_l t; m_l], \tag{21}$$

with

$$q = \exp\left(-\pi \frac{K'}{K}\right),$$

$$K = K(m) + \int_0^{\pi/2} \frac{du}{\sqrt{1 - m \sin^2 u}},$$

$$K'(m_1) = K(m), m + m_1 = 1.$$

The second term θ_{int} represents a nonlinear superposition or interaction among cnoidal waves. We write this term as

$$2\frac{d^2}{dt} \log\left[1 + \frac{F(t)}{G(t)}\right] \approx \frac{\beta_k \, cn^2(\omega t, m_k)}{1 + \gamma_k \, cn^2(\omega t, m_k)}. \tag{22}$$

If m_k take the values 0 or 1, the relation (22) is directly verified. For $0 \leq m_k \leq 1$, the relation is numerically verified with an error of $|e| \leq 5 \times 10^{-7}$. Consequently, we have

$$\theta_{nonlin} = \frac{\sum_{k=0}^{n} \beta_k \, cn^2[\eta; m_k]}{1 + \sum_{k=0}^{n} \lambda_k \, cn^2[\eta; m_k]}. \tag{23}$$

As a result, the cnoidal method yields to solutions consisting of a linear superposition and a nonlinear superposition of cnoidal waves.

Therefore, by applying the cnoidal method, the closed form solutions of the Euler angles θ, ψ and φ are obtained [43].

$$\begin{aligned} \cos \upsilon = \zeta = \zeta_2 - (\zeta_2 - \zeta_3) cn^2\left(\sqrt{\frac{|\lambda_3|}{2A}(\zeta_1 - \zeta_3)}(\xi - \xi_3), m\right) = \\ = \zeta_2 - (\zeta_2 - \zeta_3) cn^2[w(\xi - \xi_3), m], \end{aligned} \tag{24}$$

where $m = \frac{\zeta_2 - \zeta_3}{\zeta_1 - \zeta_3}$ and $w = \sqrt{\frac{|\lambda_3|}{2A}(\zeta_1 - \zeta_3)}$,

$$\begin{aligned} \psi = \frac{1}{4(A - k_1 v^2)^2 w^2} \left\{ -\frac{\beta + (C - k_2 v^2)\tau}{1 - \zeta_3} \prod\left[w(\xi - \xi_3), \frac{\zeta_2 - \zeta_3}{1 - u_3}, m\right] - \right. \\ \left. - \frac{\beta - (C - k_2 v^2)\tau}{1 + \zeta u_3} \prod\left[w(\xi - \xi_3), \frac{\zeta_2 - \zeta_3}{1 + u_3}, m\right] \right\}, \end{aligned} \tag{25}$$

$$\begin{aligned} \varphi = -\frac{\tau[C - A - (k_2 + k_1) v^2]}{A - k_1 v^2} \xi + \frac{1}{4(A - k_1 v^2)^2 w^2} \left\{ \frac{\beta + (C - k_2 v^2)\tau}{1 - \zeta_3} \times \right. \\ \left. \times \prod\left[w(\xi - \xi_3), \frac{\zeta_2 - \zeta_3}{1 - \zeta_3}, m\right] - \frac{\beta - (C - k_2 v^2)\tau}{1 + \zeta_3} \prod\left(w(\xi - \xi_3), \frac{\zeta_2 - \zeta_3}{1 + \zeta_3}, m\right) \right\}, \end{aligned} \tag{26}$$

with $\prod(x, z, m) = \int_0^x \frac{dy}{1 - z \, sn^2(y, m)}$ the normal elliptic integral of the third kind.

Functions $\zeta_1, \zeta_2, \zeta_3$ are solutions of the equation

$$\frac{1}{2}\zeta'^2 = a\zeta^3 + b\zeta^2 - a\zeta + c, \tag{27}$$

$$a = -\frac{\lambda_3}{A} \neq 0, b = \frac{1}{2A}\left(\gamma - \frac{C^2\tau^2}{A}\right), c = -\frac{1}{2A}\left(\gamma - \frac{\beta^2}{A}\right). \tag{28}$$

Our objective is to determine the functions which measure the bending of the needle (u_1 and u_2), and the torsion (u_3). To visualize the strain profile of the needle, we chose two routes (**Figure 4**). For the first route the tumor is red and the entry point is A. The second route is restricted by the presence of blood vessels that should not be touched and has the tumor (blue) with entry at point B.

Figures 5 and **6** show that the deformation of the needle for both routes. We see that the deformation is small with no tendency to chaos. The strains are described

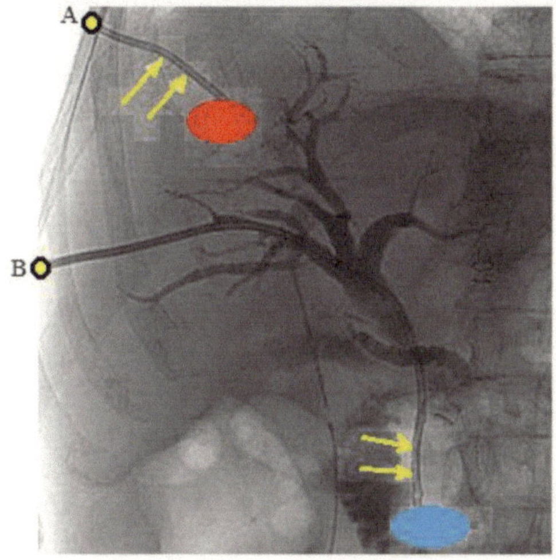

Figure 4.
Two needle trajectories: For first route the tumor is red and the entry point A, and for the second route tumor is blue and the entry point B.

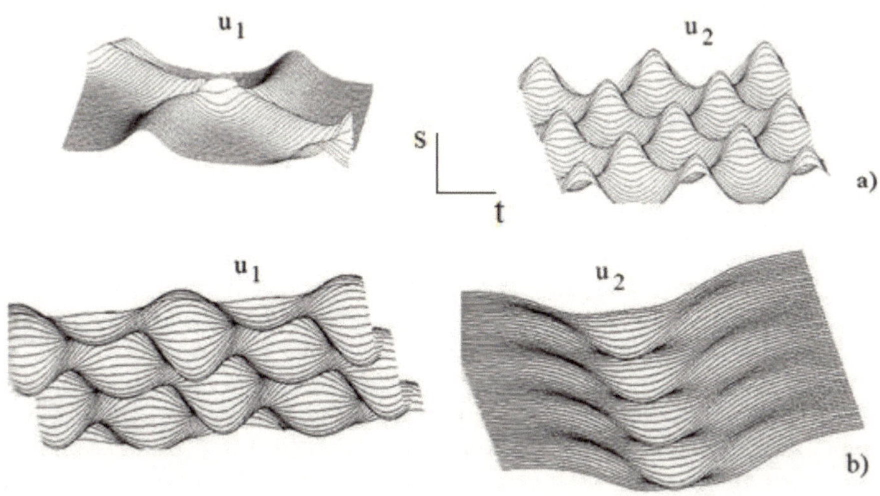

Figure 5.
Functions u_1 and u_2 for a) first route and b) second route.

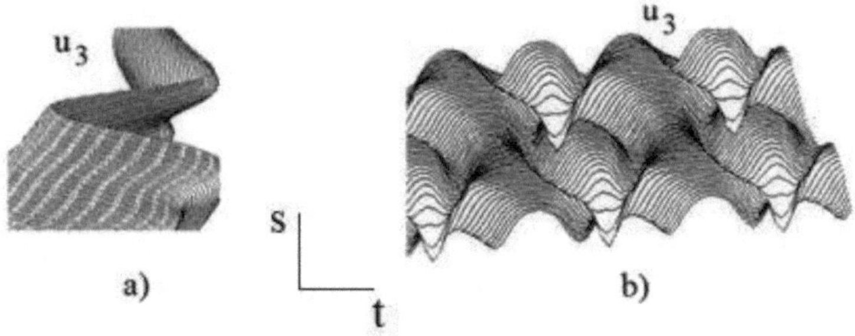

Figure 6.
Function u_3 for a) first route and b) the second route.

by localized solitons which propagate for a long time without changes. The soliton is a localized wave with an infinite number of degrees of freedom. This wave conserves its properties even after interaction with another wave. In short, this wave acts somewhat like particles [43]. The system of Eqs. (7–11) has unique properties. These properties are locally preserved such as an infinite number of exact solutions expressed in terms of the Jacobi elliptic functions or the hyperbolic functions, and the simple formulae for nonlinear superposition of explicit solutions.

3. Determination of the free-collision trajectories

Let us present a model for determining the collision-free trajectories by using the Fibonacci sequence. The trajectories are determined from the restrictions of avoiding the collisions with blood vessels, ribs and surrounding tissues, and also the interference of needles with each other. We consider that more needles are planned to be inserted into the liver [45].

The trajectory of each needle $j = 1, \ldots, n$, is defined as a set of segments connecting the insertion point with the tumor. Two binary control parameters are introduced on each needle. The first parameter is the length of the kth segment of the jth needle's trajectory, $l_{kj} = f_k/r^{kj}$, where f_k is the kth Fibonacci number and r_{kj} a scaling number. The second control parameter is the angle ω between the current needle and the previous one, $\omega \in (0, \pi)$ [46, 47].

The sequence terms in the Fibonacci problem are 1, 1, 2, 3, 5, 8, 13, 21, 34, 55, 89, 144. It is clear that each term is a sum of two preceding sequence term. In fact, the sequence can be recursively defined in the form $f_n = f_{n-1} + f_{n-2}, f_0 = 0, f_1 = 1$. The limit of the ratio of two consecutive terms in the Fibonacci string tends to the gold ratio $\varphi = (1 + \sqrt{5})/2$ [48, 49].

The Fibonacci sequence was highlighted in nature for example in the arrangement of the flower petals, in seeds and in the spiral arrangement of pine cones and pineapple. The keys on a piano are divided into Fibonacci numbers, and numerous classical compositions implement the golden section. Such an example is found in the Alleluia Choir in Handel's Messiah and in many of Chopin's preludes [50].

Development of a target drug delivery technique usually consisted of three steps. In step 1, a 2D ultrasound image of the tumor is obtained. The size and position of the tumor are analyzed by the surgeon who decides the number of required needles. In step 2, the insertion points on the skin of the needles and the positions of the targets in the tumor are established. In step 3, once the needles are placed at the target points on the skin, they are guided according to a precise surgical planning

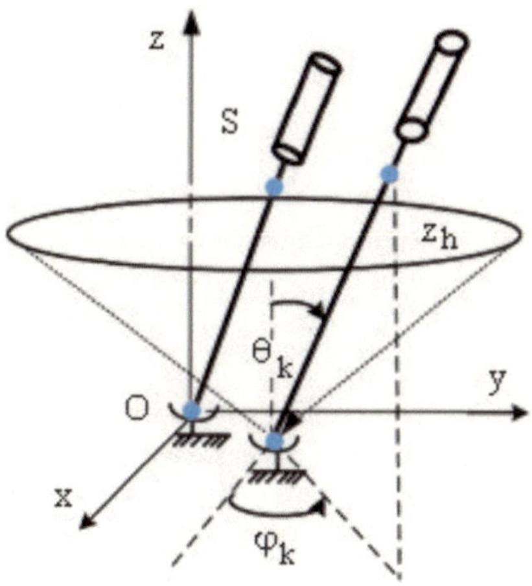

Figure 7.
The base coordinate frame.

based on the optimization of the collision-free trajectories to avoid the ribs, blood vessels and tissues in the abdominal area.

The base coordinate frame is established on the first needle with the vertical axis Oz and the origin in the insertion point (**Figure 7**). The workspace boundary for the needle is a 1D curve in each xy- plane means the z_h-plane for $z = h$, $h \in [0, h_{\max}]$ with a clinical value $h = 200$ mm. The S is the plan of the needle insertion trajectory, (θ_k, φ_k) are the rotation angles with respect to y and z axes $\theta_{\min} \leq \theta_k \leq \theta_{\max}$, $\phi_{\min} \leq \varphi_k \leq \varphi_{\max}$ [45].

The first control parameter is the length of the kth segment of the jth needle, $l_{kj} = f_k / r^{kj}$, $k = 1, \dots, m_{lk}, j = 1, \dots, n$ where f_k is the kth Fibonacci number

$$f_0 = f_1 = 1, f_{k+2} = f_{k+1} + f_k, k \geq 0. \tag{29}$$

and r_{kj} a scaling number. The second control parameter is the angle φ between the current needle and the previous one, $\varphi \in (0, \pi)$. The kinematic constraint of the jth needle, $j = 1, \dots, n$, is given by

$$\phi = \begin{bmatrix} x_j - x_{0j} - \delta_{xj} - (h - z_{0j} - \delta_{zj}) \tan\theta_j \cos\varphi_j \\ y_j - y_{0j} - y_{yj} - (h - z_{0j} - \delta_{zj}) \tan\theta_j \cos\varphi_j \end{bmatrix} = 0, \tag{30}$$

where $\left[x_{0j} + \delta_{xj}, y_{0j} + \delta_{xj}, y_{0j} + \delta_{xj}\right]^T$ is the actual target of the tip of needle $(j-1)$, $\left(\theta_j, \varphi_j\right)$ are the rotation angles with respect to y and z axes $\theta_{\min} \leq \theta_j \leq \theta_{\max}$, $\phi_{\min} \leq \varphi_j \leq \varphi_{\max}$ and $(\delta_{xj}, \delta_{yj}, \delta_{zj})$ denote the deformation of the liver.

The choice of the scaling number r_{kj} is done by a binary control

$$l_{kj} = \|x_k - x_{k-1}\| = \frac{u_{kj} f_k}{r^{kj}}. \tag{31}$$

The possible collision point between the needle and the tissue is analyzed by an identifier to check the minimum distance between needle and the surrounding tissue [45]. The minimum distance is expressed as

$$\min\left(\frac{1}{2}(r_1 - r_2)^T(r_1 - r_2)\right), \tag{32}$$

with $g_1(r_1) \leq 0$, $g_2(r_2) \leq 0$, r_1, r_2, the position vectors of two points belonging to the needle and the tissue, respectively, and g_1, g_2, the surfaces to the needle and the tissue, respectively. The interference distance or penetration is defined as

$$\min(-d), \quad g_1(r_1) \leq -\frac{d}{2}, \quad g_2(r_2) \leq -\frac{d}{2}, \tag{33}$$

where d is the penetration. The configuration of the collision-free trajectories of each needle is defined as a sequence of trajectories corresponding to a particular choice for the control (u, v). The set of all collision-free trajectories are computed based on the kinematic constraint (30) as

$$R = \left\{\sum_{k=0}^{n} \frac{u_k f_k}{r^k} \exp\left(-i\omega \sum_{j=0}^{k} v_j | (v_j) \in \{0, 1\}\right\}. \tag{34}$$

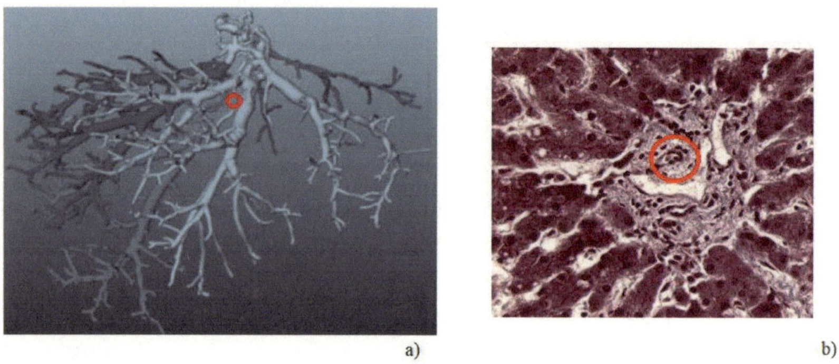

Figure 8.
a) Location of the tumor; b) tumor image seen on the microscope.

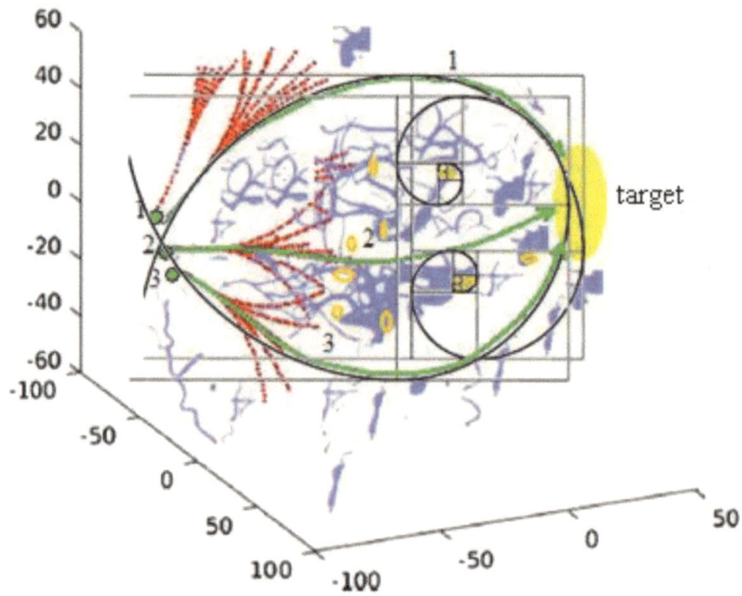

Figure 9.
Simulation of the collision-free trajectories for three-needles.

As application, the case of a tumor with a difficult location in the vicinity of the portal tree of the vascular territory in the liver, is considered (**Figure 8a**). The tumor image seen on the microscope is shown in **Figure 8b**. White and gray denote forbidden areas while the shade of purple are safe regions. The tumor is drawn in red. The Fibonacci algorithm is applied to three-needles with restrictions to avoid the collision with the tissues, blood vessels, ribs and previously inserted needles.

The task of our simulation is to determine the boundaries of each needle as a collision-free surface which represents the feasible insertion area based on given constraints. Then, the optimal trajectory of each needle can be chosen in this surface automatically.

Once all needles are placed at the predetermined epidermis and the ordering of entry is chosen to be 1, 2 and 3, following the first needle's insertion, the operation is repeated for the needles 2 and 3.

Simulation of the collision-free trajectories for three needles is presented in **Figure 9**. The insertion scheme is determined by the Fibonacci spirals. A set of free-collision trajectories (red) in the immediate vicinity of the epidermis, is suggested.

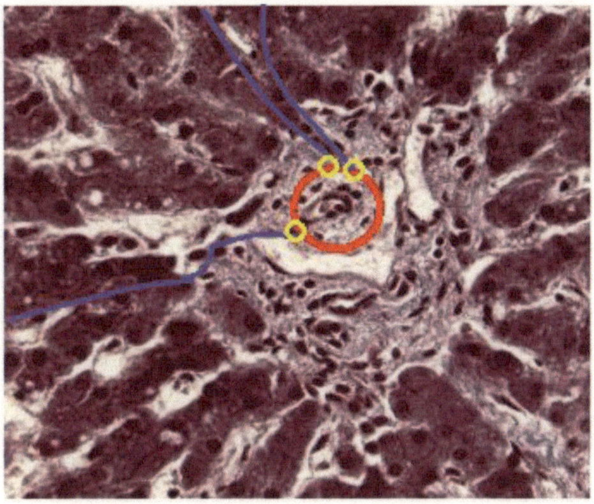

Figure 10.
Optimal solution with 3 collision-free trajectories to the target.

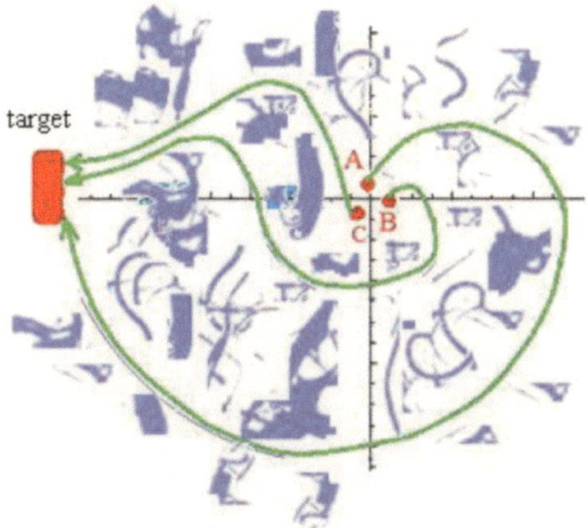

Figure 11.
Three optimal collision-free trajectories for the needle robot.

From these possible collision-free trajectories (red) the green paths corresponding to the Fibonacci spirals (black) are chosen. These trajectories avoid the blood vessels (purple) and the coasts (brown) in all directions until the tumor. Optimal solution with 3 collision-free trajectories to the target is displayed in **Figure 10**. The Fibonacci spirals with the centers in ribs (brown) are displayed for needles 1 and 3. For the needle 2, the Fibonacci.

Three locally optimal collision-free trajectories for the surgical needle corresponding to three different entry points into the skin A, B and C are displayed in **Figure 11**.

4. Conclusions

The study investigates the navigation of a flexible needle into the human liver. The role of the needle is to deliver into the tumor an active chemotherapeutic agent. The deformation of the needle during its insertion into the human liver is describe in this chapter in the context of intraoperative treatment of liver tumors based on the integrated imaging-molecular diagnosis. The needle is a bee barbed type modeled as a flexible thread within the framework of the Cosserat (micropolar) elasticity theory. The Cosserat elasticity describes the interaction between the needle and the human liver by incorporating the local rotation of points and the couple stress as well as the force stress representing the chiral properties of the human liver.

Acknowledgements

This work was supported by a grant of the Romanian ministry of Research and Innovation, CCCDI – UEFISCDI, project number PN-III-P1-1.2-PCCDI-2017-0221/ 59PCCDI/2018 (IMPROVE), within PNCDI III. We mention that *all authors have an equal contribution* to the work.

Conflict of interest

The authors of this paper certify that they have no affiliations with or involvement in any organization or entity with any financial or nonfinancial interest in the subject matter or materials discussed in this manuscript.

Author details

Veturia Chiroiu*, Ligia Munteanu, Cristian Rugină and Nicoleta Nedelcu
Institute of Solid Mechanics, Romanian Academy, Bucharest, Romania

*Address all correspondence to: veturiachiroiu@yahoo.com

References

[1] Chiroiu, V., Nedelcu, N., Munteanu, L., Rugina, C., Ionescu, M., Dragne, C., *Modeling the flexible needle insertion into the human liver,* Proceedings of the Romanian Academy, series A: Mathematics, Physics, Technical Sciences, Information Science (2020).

[2] Sahlabadi, M., Hutapea, P., *Tissue defomation and insertion force of bee-stinger inspired surgical needles*, Journal of medical device, vol.12, 034501, 1–3 (2018).

[3] Dionigi, R., *Medical Intelligence Unit: Recent Advances in Liver Surgery*, Landes Bioscience Austin, Texas (2009).

[4] Dremin, V., Potapova, E., Zherebtsov, E., Kandurova, K., Shupletsov, V., Alekseyev, A., Mamoshin, A., Dunaev A., *Optical percutaneous needle biopsy of the liver: a pilot animal and clinical study*, Scientific Reports, volume 10, Article number: 14200 (2020).

[5] Abolhassani, N., Patel, R., Moallem, M., *Control of soft tissue deformation during robotic needle insertion*, Minimally Invasive Therapy, 15(3), 165–176 (2006).

[6] Abolhassani, N., Patel, R., Moallem, M., *Needle insertion into soft tissue: A survey*, Medical Engineerings & Physics, 29, 413–431 (2007).

[7] Torzilli, G., Minagawa, M., Takayama, T., *Accurate preoperative evaluation of liver mass lesions without fine-needle biopsy,* Hepatology, 30(4), 889–893 (1999).

[8] Baker, N.E., *Emerging mechanisms of cell competition*, Nature Reviews Genetic s (2020).

[9] Petrowsky, H., Fritsch, R., Guckenberger, M., De Oliveira, M. L., Dutkowski, P., Clavien, P.A., *Modern therapeutic approaches for the treatment of malignant liver tumours*, Nature Reviews Gastroenterology & Hepatology (2020).

[10] Gino van den Bergen, *Collision detection in interactive 3D environments*, Elsevier (2004).

[11] Okamura, A.M., Simone, C., O'Leary, M.D., *Force modeling for needle insertion into soft tissue*, IEEE Trans Biomed Eng., 51,1707–16 (2004).

[12] DiMaio, S.P., Salcudean, S.E., *Needle insertion modeling and simulation*, IEEE Trans Robot Automat., 19, 864–75 (2003).

[13] DiMaio, S.P., Salcudean, S.E., *Simulated interactive needle insertion*, Proceedings of the 10th IEEE Symposium on Haptic Interfaces for Virtual Environment & Teleoperator Systems, 344–51 (2002).

[14] Maurin, B., Barbe, L., Bayle, B., Zanne, P., *In vivo study of forces during needle insertions*, Scientific Workshop on Medical Robotics, Navigation and Visualization (MRNV04), Germany, Remagen, 415–422 (2004).

[15] Lombardo, J-C, Cani, M-P, Neyret, F., *Real time collision detection for virtual surgery*, Computer Animation (CA'99), May 1999, Geneva, Switzerland, pp.82–90 (1999).

[16] Zachmann, G., *Minimal hierarchical collision detection,* Proc. ACM Symposium on Virtual Reality Software and Technology (VRST), Hong Kong, China, 121–128 (2002).

[17] Brişan, C., Boantă, C., Chiroiu, V., *Introduction in optimisation of industrial robots. Theory and applications,* Editura Academiei, Bucharest (2019).

[18] Kataoka, H., Washio, T., Audette, M., Mizuhara, K., *A model for relations*

between needle deflection, force, and thickness on needle insertion, Proceedings of the Medical Image Computing and Computer-Assisted Intervention Conference, 966–974 (2001).

[19] Pisla D., Vaida, C., Birlescu I., Nadim, A.H., Gherman, B.,Corina Radu, Plitea N., *Risk Management for the Reliability of Robotic Assisted Treatment of Non-resectable Liver Tumors*, Appl. Sci., 10(1), 52 (2020).

[20] Birlescu I., Manfred, H., Vaida C., Plitea N., Nayak A., Pisla, D., *Complete Geometric Analysis Using the Study SE(3) Parameters for a Novel, Minimally Invasive Robot Used in Liver Cancer Treatment*, Symmetry, 11(12), 1491 (2019).

[21] Vaida, C., Plitea, N., Pisla, D., Gherman, B., *Orientation module for surgical instruments - a systematical approach*, Meccanica, 48(1), 145–158 (2013).

[22] Munteanu, L., Rugină, C., Dragne, C., Chiroiu, V., *On the robotic control based on interactive activities of subjects,* Proceedings of the Romanian Academy, series A : Mathematics, Physics, Technical Sciences, Information Science, 21(1), (2020).

[23] Chiroiu, V., Munteanu, L., Ioan, R., Dragne, C., Majercsik, L., *Using the Sonification for Hardly Detectable Details in Medical Images,* Scientific Reports, 9, article number 17711 (2019).

[24] Korayem, M.H., Nikoobin, A., Azimirad, V.,*Trajectory optimization of flexible link manipulators in point-to point motion*, Robotica, 27, 825–840 (2009).

[25] Chiroiu, V., Munteanu, L., Ioan, R., Mosneguțu, V., Girip, I., *On the dL algorithm for controlling the hybrid systems*, Acta Electronica, Special Issue Proceedings of the XXIXth SISOM, 60 (1–2), 58–65, Mediamira Science Publishing (2019).

[26] Chiroiu, V., Munteanu, L., Dragne, C., Ştirbu, C., *On the diferential dynamic logic model for hybrid systems*, Acta Technica Napocensis - series: Applied Mathematics, Mechanics, and Engineering, 61(4), 2018.

[27] Majercsik, L., *On the* dL *control* applied *to a Stewart platform with flexible joints,* Romanian Journal of Mechanics, 4(1), 27–38 (2019).

[28] Motta, PM,*The three-dimensional fine structure of the liver as revealed by scanning electron microscopy*, Int. Rev. Cytol.,Suppl 6, 347–399 (1977).

[29] Ma, M.H., Biempica, L.,*The normal human liver cell*, Am. J. Pathol., 62, 353–370 (1971).

[30] Jackson RL, Morrisett JD, Gotto AM., *Lipoprotein structure and metabolism,* Physiol. Rev. 56, 259–316 (1976).

[31] Saxena, R., Theise, N.D., Crawford, J.M., *Microanatomy of the human liver-exploring the hidden interfaces*, Hepatology, 30(6), 1339–46 (1999).

[32] Si-Tayeb, K., Lemaigre, F.P., Duncan, S.A., *Organogenesis and development of the liver*, Dev. Cell.,18(2), 175–89 (2010).

[33] Yi–Je Lim, Dhanannjay Deo, Tejinde r P. Singh, Daniel B. Jones, Suvranu De, *In Situ* Measurement and Modeling of Biomechanical Response of Human Cadaveric Soft Tissues for Physics-Based Surgical Simulation, Surg Endosc., 23(6), 1298–1307 (2009).

[34] Narayan, K.S., Steele, W.J., Busch, H., *Evidence that the granular and fibrillar components of nucleoli contain 28 and 65 RNA, respectively*, Exp. Cell. Res., 43, 483–492 (1966).

[35] Habenschus, M.D., Nardini, V., Dia s, L.G., Rocha, B.A., Barbosa Jr. F. , Moraes de Oliveira, A.R., *In vitro enantioselective study of the toxicokinetic effects of chiral fungicide tebuconazole in human liver microsomes*, Ecotoxicol. Environ. Saf., 181, 96–105 (2019).

[36] Takahashi, M., Takani, D., Haba, M., Hosokawa, M., *Investigation of the chiral recognition ability of human carboxylesterase 1 using indomethacin esters*, Chirality, 32(1), 73–80 (2020).

[37] Cosserat, E., Cosserat, F., *Theorie des corps deformable*, Herman et Fils, Paris, 1909.

[38] Eringen, A.C., *Microcontinuum Field Theory*, volume II. Fluent Media, Springer, New York (2001).

[39] Eringen, A.C., Kafadar, C.B., *Polar field theories.* In A. C. Eringen,editor, Continuum Physics, volume IV, pages 1–75. Academic Press, NewYork (1976).

[40] Iesan, D., *Existence theorems in the theory of micropolar elasticity*. International Journal of Engineering Science, 8, 777–791 (1970).

[41] Iesan, D., *Existence theorems in micropolar elastostatics*, International Journal of Engineering Science, 9, 59–78 (1971).

[42] Forest, S., Sievert, R., *Nonlinear microstrain theories*, International Journal of Solids and Structures, 43(24), 7224–7245 (2006).

[43] Munteanu, L., Donescu, St., *Introduction to Soliton Theory: Applications to Mechanics,* Book Series Fundamental Theories of Physics, vol.143, Kluwer Academic Publishers, Dordrecht, Boston (Springer Netherlands) (2004).

[44] Chiroiu, V., Munteanu, L., Gliozzi, A.S., *Application of the Cosserat theory for modeling the reinforcement carbon nanotube beams*, CMC: Computers, Materials & Continua, 19(1), 1–16 (2010).

[45] Dragne, C., Chiroiu, V., Munteanu, L., Brişan, C., Rugină, C., Ioan, R., Stănescu, N-D, Stan, A.F., *On the collision free-trajectories of a multiple-needle robot based on the Fibonacci sequence,* New Trends in Mechanism and Machine Science, Volume 89 of the Mechanisms and Machine Science series, Chapter 20 pp.1–12 Springer (2019).

[46] Lai, A.C., Loreti, P., Velluci, P.: A Model for Robotic Hand Based on Fibonacci Sequence. In: Proceedings of the 11th International Conference on Informatics in Control, Automation and Robotics (ICINCO-2014), pp.577–584 (2014).

[47] Aghili, F., Parsa, K.: *Design of a reconfigurable space robot with lockable telescopic joints*. In Conference IEEE/RSJ, International Conference on Intelligent Robots and Systems (2006).

[48] Burton, D. M.: *Elementary number theory* (5th ed.). New York: McGraw-Hill (2002).

[49] Fox, W.P.: Fibonacci Search in Optimization of Unimodal Functions. Department of Mathematic Francis Marion University, Florence, SC 29501 (2002).

[50] Silverman, J. H.: *A friendly introduction to number theory*. (3rd ed.) Upper Saddle River, NJ: Pearson Education (2006)

Section 2

Microscopy Technology and Application

Chapter 3

Confocal Scanning Laser Microscopy in Medicine

Hasan Kiziltoprak, Dilara Ozkoyuncu, Kemal Tekin and Mustafa Koc

Abstract

Confocal Scanning Laser Microscopy (CSLM) offers high resolution morphological details and generates en-face images with excellent depth discrimination for visualizing different structures of the living human body non-invasively. There have been significant advances in technology since the CSLM was first defined. It has been used commonly, especially in ophthalmological area, in order to diagnose and give direction for the treatment of corneal pathologies. Ocular surface, corneal subbasal nerve plexus, filtering blebs of glaucoma surgery were also investigated widely by CSLM. With the improvements in CSLM technology over time, it is widely used in other fields than ophthalmology. The combined use of CSLM with the slit lamp biomicroscopy and optical coherence tomography will also lead to significant advances in the diagnosis and treatment of more diseases in the future.

Keywords: confocal scanning laser microscopy, laser imaging, medicine, ophthalmology, subbasal nerve plexus

1. Introduction

Confocal Scanning Laser Microscopy (CSLM) is a non-invasive imaging method for visualizing different structures of the living human body [1]. CSLM provides morphological details with high resolution and generates en-face images with excellent depth discrimination [1, 2]. CSLM is compatible with three-dimensional (3D) live imaging provided by sequential acquisition of tomograms along the depth direction [3]. There is a broad range of experimental and clinical applications on corneal analysis with CSLM. The imaging procedure may assess stromal changes in keratoconus patients [4], experimental full-thickness corneal 3D imaging [5], the quantification of morphological features of epithelial cell layers, and the subbasal nerve plexus [6–10] that has become very popular in recent years.

Since its commercialization in the late 1980's, CSLM has become one of the most applied fluorescence microscopy techniques for 3D-dimensional structural studies of biological cells and tissues [3]. Recent technological breakthroughs have led to the development of CSLM, and it has reached the current level of high resolution that can be used in many areas today. In recent years, there has been a vast increase in researchers using CSLM in many fields of medicine, especially in ophthalmology.

In this chapter, we have attempted to summarize the principles of CSLM and the application in ophthalmological and non-ophthalmological areas of medicine. Finally, it was discussed how it could give an essential direction to medical development in the future.

2. Principles of confocal scanning laser microscopy

Objects that share a conjugate focal plane are defined as with the term "confocal". In microscopic area, that means whereby the in-focus image plane can be seen from adjacent axial planes in case of coincidence between the focal plane of the objective lens and the detector. CSLM uses a diffraction-limited spot of light to illuminate the sample and an aperture in the collection light path at conjugate focus.

The first steps of CSLM were designed by Marvin Minsky in 1955 at his early education times and patented in 1957 [11]. However, there has been no significant improvement in CSLM technology over a long time as the required technologies which were either underdeveloped or non-existent at that time. Moreover, CSLM technology was new, and there was no pressing need for it by the scientific community. Therefore, the commercialization of CSLM occurred in the late 1980s. Petran *and colleagues* introduced the first tandem scanning confocal microscope in 1968 [12]. The Nipkow disk was used as the basis of a new sectioning microscope, and the field of view was achieved by simultaneously scanning multiple points on a stationary specimen using a rotating Nipkow disc. Even this allows for real-time imaging; it has the disadvantages of a very low light throughput and low image quality. In 1969, Svishchev produced the slit scanning confocal microscope based on an oscillating double-sided-mirror [13]. The Svishchev confocal microscope used two confocal adjustable slits. It was used to observe living neural tissue using an oscillating two-sided mirror for simultaneous scanning and de-scanning of the sample [13]. This design was subsequently further modified to enable real-time scanning. The slit scanning microscope was superior in tandem design in terms of shorter examining time and the requirement of low light intensity. The modern, and first commercially-successful CSLM was developed by Brad Amos and John White at the University of Cambridge. With this new technology, precise 3D visualization of ocular microstructures was achieved [14]. Modern digital image processing technology enables quantitative data to be stored noninvasively, rapidly, and with a low level of illumination.

All confocal microscopes share the same basic principle in their designs that enable optical sectioning of a relatively thick light scattering object. A directed light is crossed through an aperture and focused with the help of an objective lens onto a small area of the specimen. At each tissue location, light is reflected or backscattered and travels the same way back. It is separated from the incident beam by a beam splitter. The reflected light from that specimen was then directed onto a second aperture by a second objective lens. By this method, out-of-focus light is strongly reduced, improving image resolution and contrast considerably. The ability of this system to distinguish between light out of the focal plane yields images of higher lateral and axial resolution compared with light microscopy. As the illumination and detection paths are at the same focal plane, the term confocal is used [2, 3, 15].

The precision of CSLM is mainly based on the concept of the confocality of the investigated object with the light source and the detector plane. Such a system was limited because of its small field of view. By the time, a larger field of view obtained either by moving the specimen whereas the microscope remains stationary, or by moving the confocal system over a stationary specimen. Modern CSLM devices use the second technique. The microscope's temporal resolution determined by the speed at which a single image of the field is acquired. Poor temporal resolution is important as increased motion artifacts inevitable because of pulse, respiration, and eye movement when examining living human subjects [16].

3. Ophthalmological applications

Biological tissues usually slice with 2–5 μm thickness were cut, stained with various chemicals and examined by light transmission at high magnification as part of conventional microscopic evaluation. In ophthalmology, in vivo examination of semitransparent tissues is performed by slit lamp biomicroscopy thanks to the inventor Allvar Gullstrand [17]. With slit lamp biomicroscopy, optically cut planes are orientated sagittally and observed by a binocular microscope with the magnification up to 50-fold. However, single cell resolution is still impossible at this level of magnification. Nonetheless, a large number of corneal diseases could be diagnosed and followed up by slit lamp microscopy easily in many cases.

Since the corneal cells could not be evaluated by slit lamp biomicroscopy, CSLM has quite satisfactory use in this regard. CSLM provides the imaging of biological structures with up to a magnification of 800-fold that renders possible single cell evaluation (**Figure 1**). Secondly, the optical section is perpendicular to the slit lamp image as its direction is parallel to the corneal surface [2].

CSLM has been used in various ophthalmological conditions for corneal diagnostics. Corneal nerve degeneration and regeneration, assessment of corneal grafting and refractive surgery, contact lenses, diabetes mellitus, keratoconus, ocular surface disease, and normal anatomy are investigated by CSLM with a considerably high number of studies.

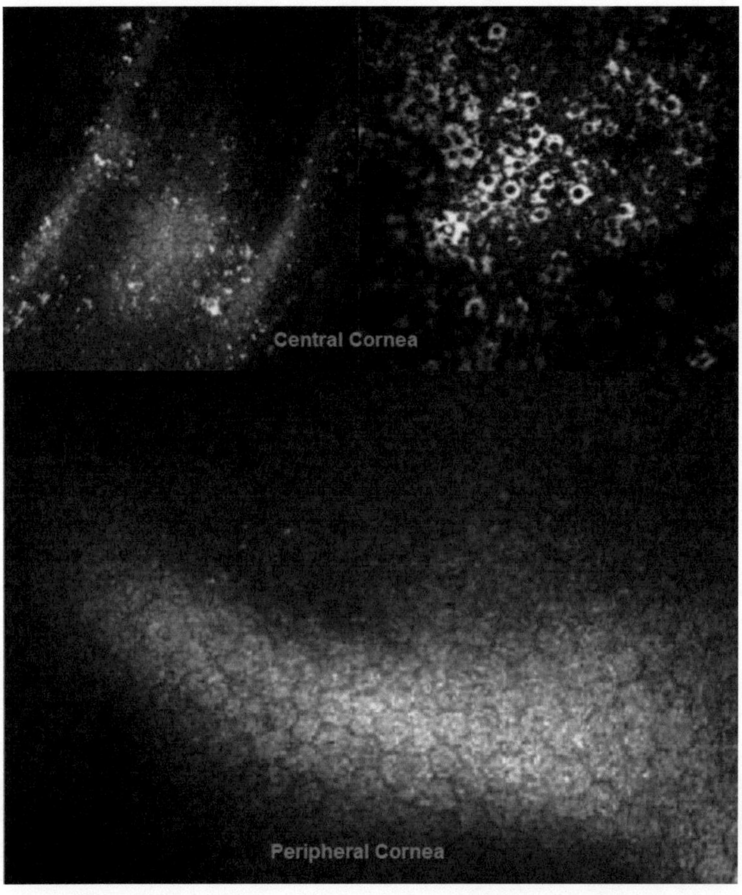

Figure 1.
Normal endothelial cells. Endothelial pigment appeared as hyper-reflective spots in some frames of the central cornea, while peripheral endothelium appeared normal. (courtesy by Mustafa Kosker).

3.1 Corneal fungal infections

Fungal keratitis can be a significant problem in especially developing countries as its slow course and treatment resistance. The clinical findings are nonspecific, and there are difficulties in diagnosis due to its delayed growth even in specific cultures. Despite their infrequent nature, in industrialized countries proper management of fungal keratitis due to prolonged diagnostic procedures ends up with devastating results [18–21]. Moreover, after initiation of antimicrobial therapy, it is still difficult to assess therapeutic response of some ulcers based upon clinical appearances by slit microscopy alone.

CSLM has been reported to be useful in diagnosis and follow up of patients in fungal keratitis [18–21]. CSLM has provided instant diagnosis without long lasting preparations of sample cultures. Also, CSLM demonstrates activated keratocytes and directly proven fungi in the corneal ulcer in differential diagnosis of non-fungal keratitis [18–21]. Although it is a rapid and noninvasive method of diagnosis of routine as well as deep-seated corneal infiltrates, its use as a primary diagnostic modality may not be possible due to its cost and limited accessibility.

3.2 Keratoconus

Keratoconus is an ectatic corneal disorder characterized by progressive thinning of cornea, which leads to an apical corneal protrusion, irregular astigmatism, superficial scar formation, and progressive decreased vision [22]. The diagnosis of keratoconus is now easy with the development of corneal topography systems. However, CSLM is another approach for the diagnosis and follow up of keratoconus. Quantitative and qualitative structural alterations were seen in all corneal layers in eyes with keratoconus, and the alterations were more prominent as the severity of disease increased [22–25].

In the keratoconus, main pathologic changes evaluated by CSLM included elongated, exfoliating superficial epithelial cells; brightly reflective material deposition within the basal epithelial cells; prominent, thickened subbasal nerves; structural changes in subbasal nerve fibers; pronounced reflectivity and irregular arrangement of stromal keratocytes; structurally abnormal anterior stromal keratocyte nuclei; folds in the anterior, mid, and posterior stroma; folds in Descemet's membrane; pleomorphism and enlargement of endothelial cells; and endothelial guttata [22]. Moreover, keratocyte density is significantly lower in subjects with keratoconus and correlated with disease severity [26]. CSLM's noninvasive nature allows the opportunity to study early microstructural changes in the keratoconic cornea and to understand its pathophysiology (**Figure 2**).

3.3 Subbasal nerve plexus

There has been an increased interest in using CSLM, that non-invasive technique as an objective diagnostic tool for peripheral neuropathies due to the capability to acquire high-resolution in vivo images of the densely innervated human cornea [27–29]. Also, the evaluation of the subbasal nerve plexus of the cornea has led to a significant rise in CSLM use to help clinicians diagnose various diseases (**Figure 3**). Morphological alterations of the corneal subbasal nerve plexus may correlate with the progression of neuropathic diseases and even predict future-incident neuropathy.

Corneal nerves are affected in cases with limbal stem cell deficiency, infection, corneal surgery, keratoconus, diabetes mellitus, lysosomal storage diseases, and keratitis [2]. Moreover, the evaluation of systemic diseases could also be possible by

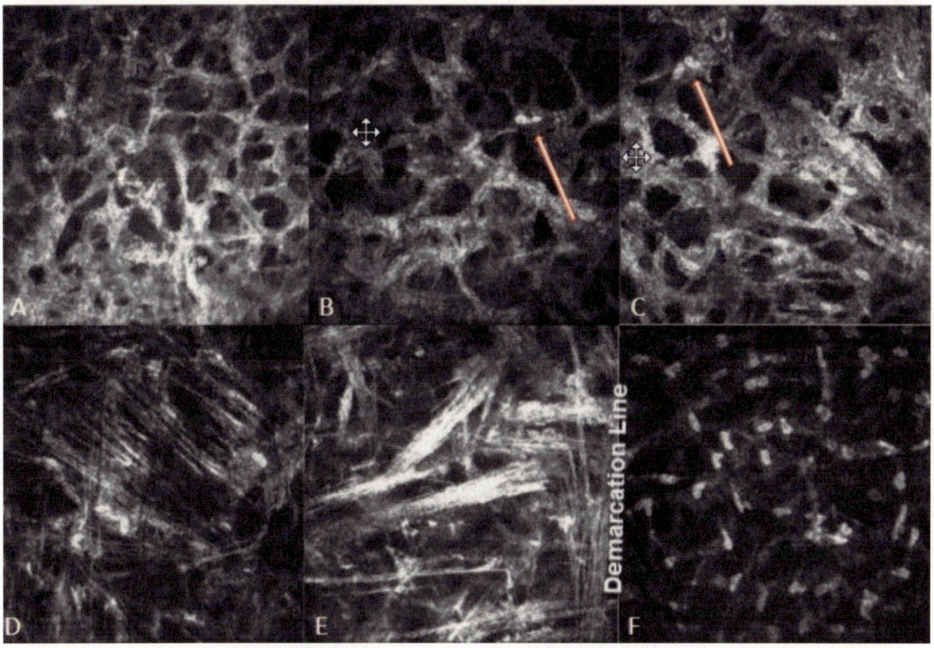

Figure 2.
Keratoconus patient that underwent corneal cross-linking treatment. Hyperreflective cytoplasm, extracellular spaces, and anterior stromal edema give a honeycomb appearance and can be observed until the 3rd month. Although almost all of the keratocytes undergo apoptosis, sporadic keratocytes are observed (arrows). Demarcation line in confocal microscopy: The long, thin, hyperreflective, needle-like structures in the middle stroma and the transition area from the wide hyperreflective stromal bands to normal keratocytes appear as the demarcation line. These hyperreflective bands can be seen in the first six months. While these changes occur in anterior stromas, there is no significant change in the keratocyte density and endothelium count behind the demarcation line. (courtesy by Mustafa Kosker).

observing corneal subbasal nerve plexus. In particular, the use of CSLM in diabetic patients, who are at risk of small fiber neuropathy leading to limb amputation, may be helpful in the early detection of small fiber neuropathy, and some preventions can be taken to slow down or eliminate the incident in both industrialized and developing countries [27].

The optical slicing of CSLM is parallel to the surface of the cornea. Therefore, it provides an ideal condition to display and to quantify structures of the subbasal nerve plexus which is located between Bowman membrane and the basal lamina of the corneal epithelial cells. It has been proposed that the imaging of the subbasal nerve plexus will be possible to find new treatment strategies and more effective prevention of serious disease.

3.4 Keratoplasty and refractive surgery

Keratoplasty is still a common method in the treatment of corneal pathologies. It has been possible because of the increase in knowledge about corneal anatomy, improvement in instruments, and advancements in technology. Today, development of modern technologies, especially in microscopy, has reached a very good position in terms of success in keratoplasty. With the widespread use of CSLM, it was possible to image a graft's microstructure as well as calculation of endothelial cell density. CSLM detected some changes such as declining of subepithelial plexus nerves, keratocytes, and endothelial cells in the central clear graft following keratoplasty [30–32]. The graft is in a stress condition which affects the normal physiological function of keratocytes and leading to the graft failure [30–32]. Activated immune

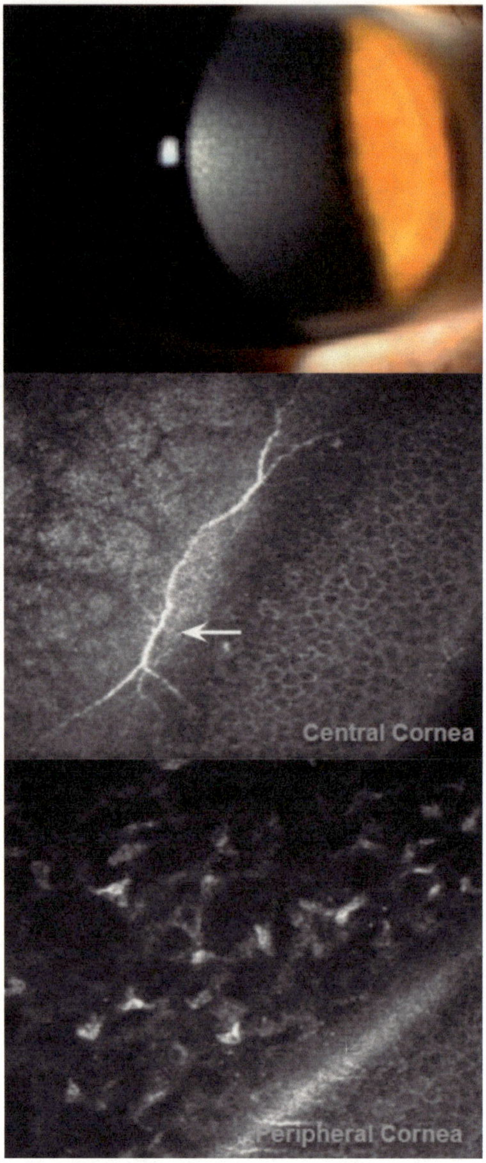

Figure 3.
Central mosaic dystrophy in a case with Megalocornea: Central cornea: The epithelium appeared normal morphologically. (white arrow): The subepithelial nerve fibers seemed to be thickened and appeared more prominent. In the stroma, starting just below Bowman's membrane, polygonal, moderately reflective areas of opacification separated by diagonal hyporeflective striations were observed. Peripheral cornea: The epithelium, bowman membrane, and anterior stroma appeared normal morphologically. (courtesy by Mustafa Kosker).

cells could also be detected in some of the clear grafts, which clearly showed that the subclinical stress of immune reaction took part in the chronic injury of the clear graft failure without any rejection episode. Therefore, morphologic alterations of corneal grafts after keratoplasty detected by CSLM enables us to be aware of corneal graft rejection and to intervene early in a possible rejection.

Refractive surgical procedures are being used frequently in the light of the increasing incidence of myopia and technological developments in refractive surgical devices. It is possible to assess the wound healing response in the living human cornea that may help in unraveling the mechanisms of corneal haze and refractive regression observed following refractive surgery. Studies are carried out in the field of CSLM in order to increase the success rate of this surgery, to detect and manage possible complications at early period [33, 34].

3.5 Contact lens

Contact lenses are used today for many different purposes. The effects of contact lenses on the eyes were evaluated with CSLM. Contact lens biocompatibility, its effects on cornea, limbal stem cells or conjunctiva, early diagnosis of devastating infections such as acanthamoeba keratitis are investigated by CSLM [35–38].

Acanthamoeba keratitis is a serious, sight-threatening corneal infection that can cause significant corneal damage and vision loss. Its incidence is on the rise because of the increasing usage of contact lenses. The diagnose of acanthamoeba keratitis is essential as its devastating nature, and CSLM can be used as an adjunct modality to the clinical data for diagnosing acanthamoeba keratitis [38].

3.6 Ocular surface diseases

CSLM has been widely used to visualize the morphology of the cornea and conjunctiva and detect changes of the ocular surface in pathological conditions such as infectious, metabolic, and trauma. The micromorphology of the corneal epithelium and stroma can be changed by infections, metabolic diseases, and genetic disorders. The progression of diseases can be observed and monitorized via CSLM [39, 40]. Chemical burns, which may result in irreversible damage to the ocular surface, constitute a large part of ocular trauma. CSLM can provide images of the goblet cells on the corneal surface which is a hallmark of limbal stem cell deficiency. The application of CSLM on chemical burns also allows for evaluation of the limbal structures and ocular surface changes after reconstructive ocular surgery [39].

Dry eye disease is another area of research for CSLM. CSLM is an effective non-invasive tool for evaluation of phenotypic alterations of the conjunctival epithelium. The use of CSLM is also crucial in the diagnosis of meibomian gland disfunction [41, 42]. It demonstrated the importance of meibomian glands for the healthy ocular surface and was also used for the effective treatment modalities of dry eye disease.

3.7 Glaucoma surgery

The formation of a filtering bleb, which attains by postoperative wound healing process, is a key factor in surgical procedures for glaucoma. Clinical and histological evaluation of these blebs has been investigated by CSLM to visualize functioning or nonfunctioning blebs at the cellular level [43, 44]. The CSLM images of filtering blebs have good consistency with the findings from previous studies. The implantation of CSLM in glaucoma surgery will be enlightened the histological processes responsible for filtration or failure.

4. Non-ophthalmological applications

CSLM is mainly improved for ocular and ocular adnexal surface structures. However, it can be suited for analyzing any surface of the human body in case of convenient for the device to reach at. On the other hand, the application of CSLM in non-transparent tissue is limited due to light-tissue interaction including reflection and refraction, absorption, and scattering of photons. In human tissues, water molecules and macromolecules such as proteins and chromophores are the main factors that affect penetration depths of the device. Therefore, CSLM images with cellular resolution can only be obtained at depths up to 300 μm [2].

CSLM has been used to evaluate the oral and pharyngeal mucosal membranes and showed promising results in dentistry applications [45–47]. Studies describing the cellular morphology and pathological alterations of the oral cavity, cervix, and esophagus also showed promising results [48, 49]. Cell morphology, tissue architecture of the epithelium, and a number of pathological skin conditions were investigated [50–52]. The amelanotic epithelial tissue of the gastrointestinal tract, lip and tongue, and the oropharynx demonstrated with CSLM [52]. CSLM identified intraepidermal blisters and acantholytic cells in pemphigus vulgaris [53]. Sinonasal inverted papilloma could also be detected noninvasively by CSLM [54]. The combination of CSLM with endoscopy is helpful in detection of schistosomiasis [55].

5. Future developments

Presently, CSLM has been a potential source of many researches and has received a high level of scientific and clinical attention in ophthalmology. Since CSLM can show high resolution images of various cellular structures within the living cornea non-invasively, it is mainly used for diagnostic purposes. However, ongoing research on this area is under development in order to improve their diagnostic potential and the usability of this technology.

5.1 Multiphoton microscopy

Corneal cell differentiation can be evaluated under various conditions by CSLM. However, the detailed information will not be satisfactory. Multiphoton microscopy, which uses a non-linear interaction mechanism, can be more useful for evaluation of cellular morphology [2]. According to multiphoton absorption, the background signal is strongly suppressed and leads to an increased penetration depth for this technique [56]. Multiphoton microscopy can be a superior alternative to confocal microscopy due to its deeper tissue penetration, efficient light detection, and reduced photobleaching. Multiphoton microscopy is reported as a promising technique for non-invasive detection of diabetic neuropathy [56, 57]. Information derived from this technology may help to develop new drugs for the treatment of diabetic neuropathy.

5.2 Slit lamp microscopy on a cellular level using CSLM

Slit lamp microscopy is a revolution for ophthalmology. Despite whole anterior segment structures can be evaluated clinically, information on cellular level cannot be attained. Recently, an in vivo method for 3D volumetric reconstruction of the cornea on a cellular level with volume sizes up to around 250 × 300 × 400 μm^3 has been reported. [58]. A piezo actuator is implanted to the microscope objective for image acquisition. Moreover, the automated, closed-loop control of the focal plane enables fast and precise focus positioning. Additionally, a novel contact cap with a concave surface has been presented that reduced eye movements by up to 87%. Therefore, the cuboid volume of the generated 3D reconstruction significantly increased. The possibility to generate oblique sections using isotropic volume stacks opened the window to slit lamp microscopy on a cellular level. The diagnosis can be made at cellular level during examination, and the treatment of diseases can be planned more effectively with the widespread useage of this technology,

5.3 Optical coherence tomography guided CSLM

CSLM is valuable for studying corneal morphology at cellular level non-invasively. However, certain drawbacks such as small field of view limit its usability. The exact CSLM image location and orientation inside the cornea are difficult to locate. Therefore, a combination with optical coherence tomography (OCT) was adapted to the conventional CSLM in order to overcome this limitation.

The combination of both technologies renders it possible to track image position and orientation in real-time [2, 59]. Real-time evaluation of CSLM image plane position and its orientation within the cornea through the OCT section provides an enhanced location-based diagnosis. It is now possible to specify the angle between the corneal surface and the image. Further studies will be necessary for optimizing the system design and OCT scan patterns. In the future, the combination of these technologies will be used widely for diagnostic purposes and will give direction to the treatment.

6. Conclusion

CSLM allows ocular structures and ocular surfaces to be assessed at cellular level. 2D tessellation or 3D reconstruction of the ophthalmic as well as non-ophthalmic tissue evaluation is possible. This technology is still promising, and close and direct collaboration between clinical science and basic science as well as industry partners can help it to reach its potential. CSLM's combination with several other technologies will also affect our understanding of diseases, diagnosis, and treatment options in the near future.

Acknowledgements

The authors thank to Assoc Prof. Dr. Mustafa Kosker from Ophthalmology Clinic of Health Sciences University Dışkapı Yıldırım Beyazıt Training and Researsch Hospital for sharing his valuable work in the field of CSLM with them.

Funding

No funding was received for this research.

Conflict of interest

All authors certify that they have no affiliations with or involvement in any organization or entity with any financial interest (such as honoraria; educational grants; participation in speakers' bureaus; membership, employment, consultancies, stock ownership, or other equity interest; and expert testimony or patent-licensing arrangements), or non-financial interest (such as personal or professional relationships, affiliations, knowledge or beliefs) in the subject matter or materials discussed in this manuscript.

Author details

Hasan Kiziltoprak[1*], Dilara Ozkoyuncu[2], Kemal Tekin[3] and Mustafa Koc[4]

1 FEBO, FICO, Bingol Maternity and Child Diseases Hospital, Ophthalmology Department, Bingol, Turkey

2 FEBO, Bilecik Training and Research Hospital, Ophthalmology Department, Bilecik, Turkey

3 Ophthalmology Department, Hatay Mustafa Kemal University, Hatay, Turkey

4 Kayseri Mayagoz Hospital, Kayseri, Turkey

*Address all correspondence to: hsnkzltprk21@gmail.com

References

[1] Patel DV, McGhee CN. Contemporary in vivo confocal microscopy of the living human cornea using white light and laser scanning techniques: a major review. Clin Exp Ophthalmol. 2007;35(1):71-88 doi: 10.1111/j.1442-9071.2007.01423.x.

[2] Stachs O, Guthoff RF, Aumann S. In Vivo Confocal Scanning Laser Microscopy. 2019 Aug 14. In: Bille JF, editor. High Resolution Imaging in Microscopy and Ophthalmology: New Frontiers in Biomedical Optics [Internet]. Cham (CH): Springer; 2019. Chapter 12. PMID: 32091848.

[3] Bayguinov PO, Oakley DM, Shih CC, Geanon DJ, Joens MS, Fitzpatrick JAJ. Modern Laser Scanning Confocal Microscopy. Curr Protoc Cytom. 2018 ;85(1):e39. doi: 10.1002/cpcy.39.,

[4] Mazzotta C, Balestrazzi A, Traversi C, Baiocchi S, Caporossi T, Tommasi C, Caporossi A. Treatment of progressive keratoconus by riboflavin-UVA-induced cross-linking of corneal collagen: ultrastructural analysis by Heidelberg Retinal Tomograph II in vivo confocal microscopy in humans. Cornea. 2007 ;26(4):390-7. doi: 10.1097/ICO.0b013e318030df5a.

[5] Petroll WM, Weaver M, Vaidya S, McCulley JP, Cavanagh HD. Quantitative 3-dimensional corneal imaging in vivo using a modified HRT-RCM confocal microscope. Cornea. 2013;32(4):e36-43. doi: 10.1097/ICO.0b013e31825ec44e.

[6] Shetty R, Deshmukh R, Shroff R, Dedhiya C, Jayadev C. Subbasal Nerve Plexus Changes in Chronic Migraine. Cornea. 2018;37(1):72-75. doi: 10.1097/ICO.0000000000001403.

[7] Garcia-Gonzalez M, Cañadas P, Gros-Otero J, Rodriguez-Perez I, Cañones-Zafra R, Kozobolis V, Teus MA. Long-term corneal subbasal nerve plexus regeneration after laser in situ keratomileusis. J Cataract Refract Surg. 2019;45(7):966-971. doi: 10.1016/j.jcrs.2019.02.019

[8] Flockerzi E, Daas L, Seitz B. Structural changes in the corneal subbasal nerve plexus in keratoconus. Acta Ophthalmol. 2020;98(8):e928-e932. doi: 10.1111/aos.14432.

[9] Allgeier S, Maier S, Mikut R, Peschel S, Reichert KM, Stachs O, Köhler B. Mosaicking the subbasal nerve plexus by guided eye movements. Invest Ophthalmol Vis Sci. 2014;55(9):6082-9. doi: 10.1167/iovs.14-14698.

[10] Köhler B, Allgeier S, Eberle F, Maier S, Peschel S, Reichert KM, Stachs O. Großflächige Abbildung kornealer Nervenfasern durch geführte Augenbewegungen [Large-scale imaging of corneal nerve fibres by guided eye movements]. Klin Monbl Augenheilkd. 2014;231(12):1170-3. doi: 10.1055/s-0034-1383331.

[11] Minsky M. Memoir on inventing the confocal scanning microscope. *Scanning*, 1988; *10*: 128-138. doi: 10.1002/sca.4950100403

[12] Petran M, Hadravsky M, Egger MD, Galambos R. Tandem scanning reflected-light microscope. *J Opt Soc Am* 1968; **58**: 661-4.

[13] Svishchev GM. Microscope for the study of transparent lightscattering objects in incident light. *Opt Spectrosc* 1969; 30: 188-91

[14] White JG, AmosWB. Confocal microscopy comes of age. *Nature* 1987; 328, 183-184. doi: 10.1038/328183a0.

[15] Guthoff RF, Baudouin C, Stave J. Atlas of Confocal Laser Scanning

In-vivo Microscopy in Opthalmology Principles and Applications in Diagnostic and Therapeutic Ophtalmology. Springer, 2006.

[16] Patel DV, McGhee CN. Contemporary in vivo confocal microscopy of the living human cornea using white light and laser scanning techniques: a major review. Clin Exp Ophthalmol. 2007;35(1):71-88. doi: 10.1111/j.1442-9071.2007.01423.x

[17] Timoney PJ, Breathnach CS. Allvar Gullstrand and the slit lamp 1911. Ir J Med Sci. 2013;182(2):301-5. doi: 10.1007/s11845-012-0873-y.

[18] Chidambaram JD, Prajna NV, Palepu S, Lanjewar S, Shah M, Elakkiya S, Lalitha P, Macleod D, Burton MJ. Cellular morphological changes detected by laser scanning in vivo confocal microscopy associated with clinical outcome in fungal keratitis. Sci Rep. 2019 ;9(1):8334. doi: 10.1038/s41598-019-44833-9.

[19] Kheirkhah A, Syed ZA, Satitpitakul V, Goyal S, Müller R, Tu EY, Dana R. Sensitivity and Specificity of Laser-Scanning In Vivo Confocal Microscopy for Filamentous Fungal Keratitis: Role of Observer Experience. Am J Ophthalmol. 2017; 179:81-89. doi: 10.1016/j.ajo.2017.04.011.

[20] Wang YE, Tepelus TC, Vickers LA, Baghdasaryan E, Gui W, Huang P, Irvine JA, Sadda S, Hsu HY, Lee OL. Role of in vivo confocal microscopy in the diagnosis of infectious keratitis. Int Ophthalmol. 2019;39(12):2865-2874. doi: 10.1007/s10792-019-01134-4.

[21] Vaddavalli PK, Garg P, Sharma S, Sangwan VS, Rao GN, Thomas R. Role of confocal microscopy in the diagnosis of fungal and acanthamoeba keratitis. Ophthalmology. 2011;118(1):29-35. doi: 10.1016/j.ophtha.2010.05.018.

[22] Uçakhan OO, Kanpolat A, Ylmaz N, Ozkan M. In vivo confocal microscopy findings in keratoconus. Eye Contact Lens. 2006;32(4):183-91. doi: 10.1097/01.icl.0000189038.74139.4a. PMID: 16845264.

[23] Ku JY, Niederer RL, Patel DV, Sherwin T, McGhee CN. Laser scanning in vivo confocal analysis of keratocyte density in keratoconus. Ophthalmology. 2008;115(5):845-50. doi: 10.1016/j.ophtha.2007.04.067.

[24] Song P, Wang S, Zhang P, Sui W, Zhang Y, Liu T, Gao H. The Superficial Stromal Scar Formation Mechanism in Keratoconus: A Study Using Laser Scanning In Vivo Confocal Microscopy. Biomed Res Int. 2016;2016:7092938. doi: 10.1155/2016/7092938.

[25] Götze A, von Keyserlingk S, Peschel S, Jacoby U, Schreiver C, Köhler B, Allgeier S, Winter K, Röhlig M, Jünemann A, Guthoff R, Stachs O, Fischer DC. The corneal subbasal nerve plexus and thickness of the retinal layers in pediatric type 1 diabetes and matched controls. Sci Rep. 2018;8(1):14. doi: 10.1038/s41598-017-18284-z.

[26] Niederer RL, Perumal D, Sherwin T, McGhee CN. Laser scanning in vivo confocal microscopy reveals reduced innervation and reduction in cell density in all layers of the keratoconic cornea. Invest Ophthalmol Vis Sci. 2008;49(7):2964-70.

[27] Allgeier S, Bartschat A, Bohn S, Peschel S, Reichert KM, Sperlich K, Walckling M, Hagenmeyer V, Mikut R, Stachs O, Köhler B. 3D confocal laser-scanning microscopy for large-area imaging of the corneal subbasal nerve plexus. Sci Rep. 2018;8(1):7468. doi: 10.1038/s41598-018-25915-6.

[28] De Silva MEH, Zhang AC, Karahalios A, Chinnery HR, Downie LE. Laser scanning in vivo confocal microscopy (IVCM) for evaluating human corneal sub-basal nerve plexus parameters: protocol

for a systematic review. BMJ Open. 2017;7(11):e018646. doi: 10.1136/bmjopen-2017-018646.

[29] Koschmieder A, Stachs O, Kragl B, Stahnke T, Sterenczak KA, Henze L, Jünemann AG, Junghanss C, Guthoff RF, Murua Escobar H. Non-invasive detection of corneal sub-basal nerve plexus changes in multiple myeloma patients by confocal laser scanning microscopy. Biosci Rep. 2020;40(10):BSR20193563. doi: 10.1042/BSR20193563.

[30] Wang D, Song P, Wang S, Sun D, Wang Y, Zhang Y, Gao H. Laser Scanning In Vivo Confocal Microscopy of Clear Grafts after Penetrating Keratoplasty. Biomed Res Int. 2016;2016:5159746. doi: 10.1155/2016/5159746.

[31] Niederer RL, Perumal D, Sherwin T, McGhee CN. Corneal innervation and cellular changes after corneal transplantation: an in vivo confocal microscopy study. Invest Ophthalmol Vis Sci. 2007;48(2):621-6. doi: 10.1167/iovs.06-0538.

[32] Szaflik JP, Kaminska A, Udziela M, Szaflik J. In vivo confocal microscopy of corneal grafts shortly after penetrating keratoplasty. Eur J Ophthalmol. 2007;17(6):891-6. doi: 10.1177/112067210701700604.

[33] Erie JC, Hodge DO, Bourne WM. Confocal microscopy evaluation of stromal ablation depth after myopic laser in situ keratomileusis and photorefractive keratectomy. J Cataract Refract Surg. 2004;30(2):321-5. doi: 10.1016/j.jcrs.2003.09.058.

[34] Gokmen F, Jester JV, Petroll WM, McCulley JP, Cavanagh HD. In vivo confocal microscopy through-focusing to measure corneal flap thickness after laser in situ keratomileusis. J Cataract Refract Surg. 2002;28(6):962-70. doi: 10.1016/s0886-3350(02)01275-0.

[35] Ghosh S, Mutalib HA, Sharanjeet-Kaur, Ghoshal R, Retnasabapathy S. Effects of contact lens wearing on keratoconus: a confocal microscopy observation. Int J Ophthalmol. 2017;10(2):228-234. doi: 10.18240/ijo.2017.02.08.

[36] Jalbert I, Rejab S. Increased numbers of Demodex in contact lens wearers. Optom Vis Sci. 2015;92(6):671-8. doi: 10.1097/OPX.0000000000000605.

[37] Bantseev V, McCanna DJ, Driot JY, Ward KW, Sivak JG. Biocompatibility of contact lens solutions using confocal laser scanning microscopy and the in vitro bovine cornea. Eye Contact Lens. 2007;33(6 Pt 1):308-16. doi: 10.1097/ICL.0b013e31803c55ad.

[38] Kheirkhah A, Satitpitakul V, Syed ZA, Müller R, Goyal S, Tu EY, Dana R. Factors Influencing the Diagnostic Accuracy of Laser-Scanning In Vivo Confocal Microscopy for Acanthamoeba Keratitis. Cornea. 2018 ;37(7):818-823. doi: 10.1097/ICO.0000000000001507.

[39] Wang Y, Le Q, Zhao F, Hong J, Xu J, Zheng T, Sun X. Application of in vivo laser scanning confocal microscopy for evaluation of ocular surface diseases: lessons learned from pterygium, meibomian gland disease, and chemical burns. Cornea. 2011;30 Suppl 1:S25-8. doi: 10.1097/ICO.0b013e318227fcd9.

[40] Falke K, Prakasam RK, Hovakimyan M, Zhivov A, Guthoff RF, Stachs O. Oberflächenerkrankungen des Auges unterschiedlicher Genese - klinische und konfokalmikroskopische Untersuchungen [Pathological conditions of the ocular surface -- a clinical and confocal laser-scanning microscopy study]. Klin Monbl Augenheilkd. 2013;230(1):59-63. German. doi: 10.1055/s-0032-1327947.

[41] Kojima T, Matsumoto Y, Dogru M, Tsubota K. The application of in vivo laser scanning confocal microscopy as a

tool of conjunctival in vivo cytology in the diagnosis of dry eye ocular surface disease. Mol Vis. 2010;16:2457-64.

[42] Iaccheri B, Torroni G, Cagini C, Fiore T, Cerquaglia A, Lupidi M, Cillino S, Dua HS. Corneal confocal scanning laser microscopy in patients with dry eye disease treated with topical cyclosporine. Eye (Lond). 2017;31(5):788-794. doi: 10.1038/eye.2017.3.

[43] Sbeity Z, Palmiero PM, Tello C, Liebmann JM, Ritch R. Noncontact in vivo scanning laser microscopy of filtering blebs. J Glaucoma. 2009;18(6):479-83. doi: 10.1097/IJG.0b013e31818d38bf.

[44] DI Staso S, Agnifili L, DI Gregorio A, Climastone H, Galassi E, Fasanella V, Ciancaglini M. Three-dimensional Laser Scanning Confocal Analysis of Conjunctival Microcysts in Glaucomatous Patients Before and After Trabeculectomy. In Vivo. 2017;31(6):1081-1088. doi: 10.21873/invivo.11173.

[45] El Hachem R, Khalil I, Le Brun G, Pellen F, Le Jeune B, Daou M, El Osta N, Naaman A, Abboud M. Dentinal tubule penetration of AH Plus, BC Sealer and a novel tricalcium silicate sealer: a confocal laser scanning microscopy study. Clin Oral Investig. 2019;23(4):1871-1876. doi: 10.1007/s00784-018-2632-6.

[46] White WM, Rajadhyaksha M, González S, Fabian RL, Anderson RR. Noninvasive imaging of human oral mucosa in vivo by confocal reflectance microscopy. Laryngoscope. 1999;109(10):1709-17. doi: 10.1097/00005537-199910000-00029.

[47] Inoue H, Igari T, Nishikage T, Ami K, Yoshida T, Iwai T. A novel method of virtual histopathology using laser-scanning confocal microscopy in-vitro with untreated fresh specimens from the gastrointestinal mucosa. Endoscopy. 2000;32(6):439-43. doi: 10.1055/s-2000-654.

[48] Just T, Stave J, Boltze C, Wree A, Kramp B, Guthoff RF, Pau HW. Laser scanning microscopy of the human larynx mucosa: a preliminary, ex vivo study. Laryngoscope. 2006;116(7):1136-41. doi: 10.1097/01.mlg.0000217529.53079.59.

[49] Drezek RA, Collier T, Brookner CK, Malpica A, Lotan R, Richards-Kortum RR, Follen M. Laser scanning confocal microscopy of cervical tissue before and after application of acetic acid. Am J Obstet Gynecol. 2000;182(5):1135-9. doi: 10.1067/mob.2000.104844.

[50] Fuchs C, Ortner VK, Hansen FS, Philipsen PA, Haedersdal M. Subclinical effects of adapalene-benzoyl peroxide: a prospective in vivo imaging study on acne micromorphology and transfollicular delivery. J Eur Acad Dermatol Venereol. 2021 Jan 28. doi: 10.1111/jdv.17140.

[51] González S, et al. Characterization of psoriasis in vivo by reflectance confocal microscopy. J Med. 1999;30(5-6):337-56.

[52] Busam KJ, Charles C, Lee G, Halpern AC. Morphologic features of melanocytes, pigmented keratinocytes, and melanophages by in vivo confocal scanning laser microscopy. Mod Pathol. 2001;14(9):862-8. doi: 10.1038/modpathol.3880402

[53] Bağcı IS, Aoki R, Vladimirova G, Sárdy M, Ruzicka T, French LE, Hartmann D. Simultaneous immunofluorescence and histology in pemphigus vulgaris using ex vivo confocal laser scanning microscopy. J Biophotonics. 2021 Jan 24. doi: 10.1002/jbio.202000509.

[54] Óvári A, Starke N, Schuldt T, Schröder S, Zonnur S, Erbersdobler A,

Lankenau E, Stachs O, Just T, Mlynski R, Olzowy B. Optical coherence tomography and confocal laser scanning microscopy as non-invasive tools in the diagnosis of sinonasal inverted papilloma: a pilot study. Eur Arch Otorhinolaryngol. 2018;275(7):1775-1781. doi: 10.1007/s00405-018-4995-3.

[55] Holtfreter MC, Stachs O, Reichard M, Loebermann M, Guthoff RF, Reisinger EC. Confocal laser scanning microscopy for detection of *Schistosoma mansoni* eggs in the gut of mice. PLoS One. 2011;6(4):e18799. doi: 10.1371/journal.pone.0018799.

[56] Ehmke T, Leckelt J, Reichard M, Weiss H, Hovakimyan M, Heisterkamp A, Stachs O, Baltrusch S. In vivo nonlinear imaging of corneal structures with special focus on BALB/c and streptozotocin-diabetic Thy1-YFP mice. Exp Eye Res. 2016;146:137-44. doi: 10.1016/j.exer.2015.11.024.

[57] Bueno JM, Cruz-Castillo R, Avilés-Trigueros M, Bautista-Elivar N. Arrangement of the photoreceptor mosaic in a diabetic rat model imaged with multiphoton microscopy. Biomed Opt Express. 2020;11(9):4901-4914. doi: 10.1364/BOE.399835.

[58] Bohn S, Sperlich K, Allgeier S, Bartschat A, Prakasam R, Reichert KM, Stolz H, Guthoff R, Mikut R, Köhler B, Stachs O. Cellular *in vivo* 3D imaging of the cornea by confocal laser scanning microscopy. Biomed Opt Express. 2018;9(6):2511-2525. doi: 10.1364/BOE.9.002511.

[59] Iftimia N, Yélamos O, Chen CJ, Maguluri G, Cordova MA, Sahu A, Park J, Fox W, Alessi-Fox C, Rajadhyaksha M. Handheld optical coherence tomography-reflectance confocal microscopy probe for detection of basal cell carcinoma and delineation of margins. J Biomed Opt. 2017;22(7):76006. doi: 10.1117/1.JBO.22.7.076006.

Chapter 4

Cornea Confocal Microscopy: Utilities and Perspectives

Eduardo Rojas Alvarez

Abstract

The cornea is the ocular refractive medium with the greatest refractive power of the eye. The study of it is of vital importance for the diagnosis and follow-up of ophthalmological diseases with the aim of achieving high standards of visual acuity in our patients. Confocal microscopy of the cornea allows in-depth study of it, quickly, safely, painlessly, obtaining high-resolution images of the corneal sublayers. This chapter summarizes the procedure for performing corneal confocal microscopy, the normal characteristics of the tissue with real images of our patients, as well as a brief explanation of the main applications of this technology in the study of corneal dystrophies (keratoconus), in refractive surgery, corneal transplantation, infectious keratitis, glaucoma filtration bulla, among other topics.

Keywords: microscopía confocal, cornea, epitelio, estroma, endotelio

1. Introduction

The sense of vision is one of the most precious, the study of the visual phenomenon has always been in the sights of researchers at all times, with the common goal of finding the necessary tools to diagnose and treat ophthalmological disorders in a timely manner and therefore, achieve better results of visual acuity in patients.

Within the eyeball, one of the most important anatomical elements in terms of visual contribution is the cornea. This tissue is part of the outermost layer of the eyeball, it is made up of 5 layers, has a thickness in the central part of 0.5 mm and is thicker in the peripheral part. It is avascular and confers most of the ocular diopter power.In ophthalmology consultations, corneal diseases are a frequent reason for consultation, since they are the cause of decreased visual acuity. There are different diagnostic methods used by the ophthalmologist to study the cornea, such as: anterior biomicroscope, corneal topography, fluorescein staining, endothelial microscopy, keratometry, among others.

The advent of confocal microscopy has made it possible to study the corneal sublayers in greater depth, in vivo, without discomfort and with rapid obtaining of high resolution images. The principle of confocality has been very useful for the study of corneal dystrophies, patients with corneal refractive surgery, corneal infections, contact lens users, corneal transplantation, among other applications. All these results have positioned confocal microscopy as a method of great diagnostic importance in the study of the human cornea, aspects that we will summarize in the current chapter.

IntechOpen

2. Development

2.1 General principles of cornea confocal microscopy

Until recently, the diagnosis of diseases of the cornea and the ocular surface has been based on the traditional anterior biomicroscopy. The exponential evolution of technology that has occurred in the last two decades has been led by the introduction of new instruments such as corneal topography, ultrasonic biomicroscopy and optical coherence tomography, among others, for the analysis of the ocular anterior segment [1–3].

These techniques offer details of the corneal curvature or macroscopic sections for the examination of structures. On the other hand, the microscopic morphology of the ocular surface was only performed by ex vivo histology, which presents limitations such as tissue degeneration, the presence of artifacts and the impossibility of evaluating the processes of disease.

Confocal microscopy is a non-invasive method for the study of microscopic images in living tissues, which has been used for the investigation of corneal microstructure since the beginning of the 1990s [4–6]. The study of images has evolved from experimental levels in laboratory research, to applications in healthy and sick patients [7, 8].

The confocal microscope for the study of cells of the nervous system in vivo, original from 1955, it was developed by Minsky in 1988. This allowed optical theory to be more formally developed and extended in the years of that decade (Wilson and Sheppard, 1984) and in the following decade (Hill; Masters and Thaer, 1994) [9, 10]. The basic principle of confocal microscopy is that an isolated point of tissue can be illuminated by a beam of light and simultaneously captured by a camera in the same plane. This produces a high resolution image [7, 10–13].

Currently, there are several types of confocal microscopes, for example: the Confoscan P4 (Tomey, United States), the Confoscan 4 (Nidek, Japan) and the confocal corneal laser microscope (Heidelberg Retina Tomograph II Rostock Corneal Module: HRTII) (Heidelberg, Germany), among others [3, 14, 15].

All confocal microscopes have the same basic principles of operation.8, 10 Light passes through an aperture and is focused on an objective lens in a small area. Light is reflected from this area and passes through a second objective lens. This light is focused on a second aperture, the out-of-focus light is eliminated. Illumination and detection are in the same focal plane, therefore the term confocal is used [10, 16–19].

The system has the ability to discriminate high-resolution lateral and axial images of light that is not in the focal plane, compared to light microscopes. Clearly as a system it is limited by a small field view. Image quality generally depends on two factors: contrast and resolution. It also depends on the numerical aperture of the objective lens, illumination levels, and the reflectivity of the studied structures and the wavelength of the illumination source [8, 14] (**Figures 1** and **2**).

2.2 The normal cornea by confocal microscopy

The superficial epithelium of the cornea is observed as hexagonal cells with bright edges with a defined nucleus and homogeneous cytoplasm [20–22]. The cells have a characteristic polygonal shape, almost hexagonal, which are characterized by a highly reflective cytoplasm since they are in a high continuous flaking process, with a shiny core and space perinuclear dark clearly visible. The superficial epithelium is five microns thick [11, 22–26] (**Figure 3**).

Intermediate stratum cells are characterized by bright edges and dark cytoplasm. The nucleus can be distinguished with great difficulty [27–29]. The average density

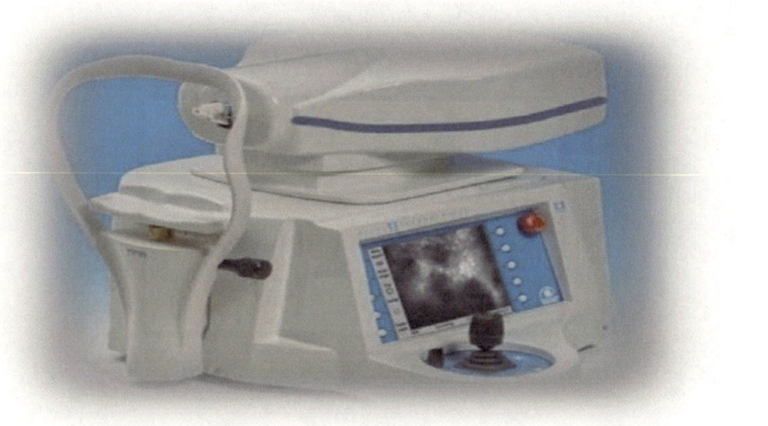

Figure 1.
NIDEK ConfoScan 4 confocal microscope.

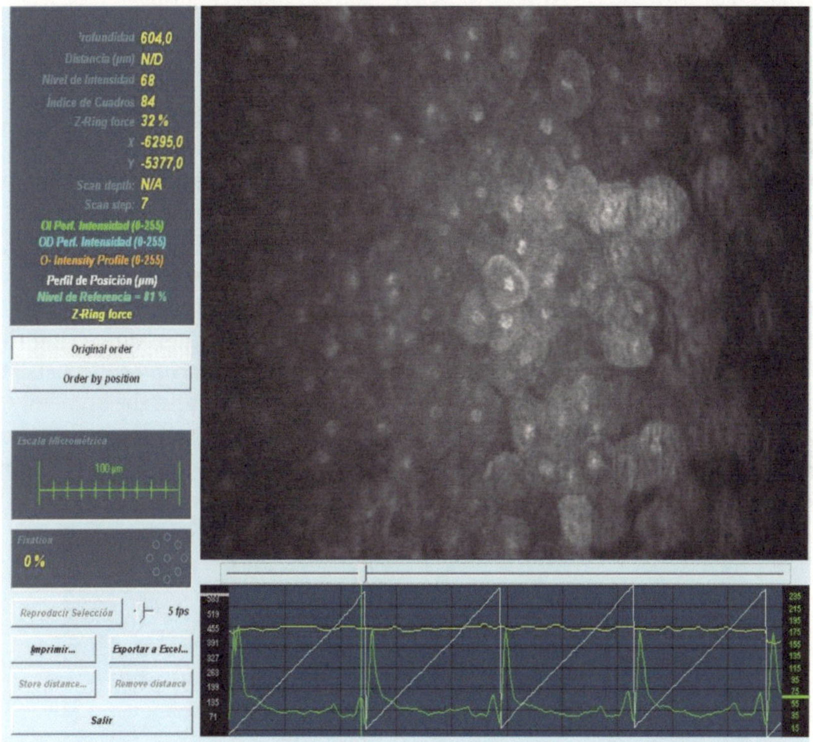

Figure 2.
Full focus quantitative confocal microscopy (CMTF), where the selected image is seen in the upper right: Apical epithelium one year after LASIK. The top left shows the parameters of depth, distance, intensity level, pressure of the Z ring, among others.

is approximately 5000 cells/mm^2 in the central cornea and 5,500 cells/mm^2 in the periphery. The cells of the middle stratum have the lowest reflectivity in the entire corneal epithelium [12, 22, 30, 31].

The basal cells are located immediately above Bowman's membrane. They present bright cell borders in which the nucleus is not visible [7, 12, 23, 32–34]. Comparison between cells reveals inhomogeneous reflectivity of the cytoplasm. Like the cells of the intermediate stratum, basal cells show only minimal variation in their shape and size. In terms of cell density in normal subjects, the ratio

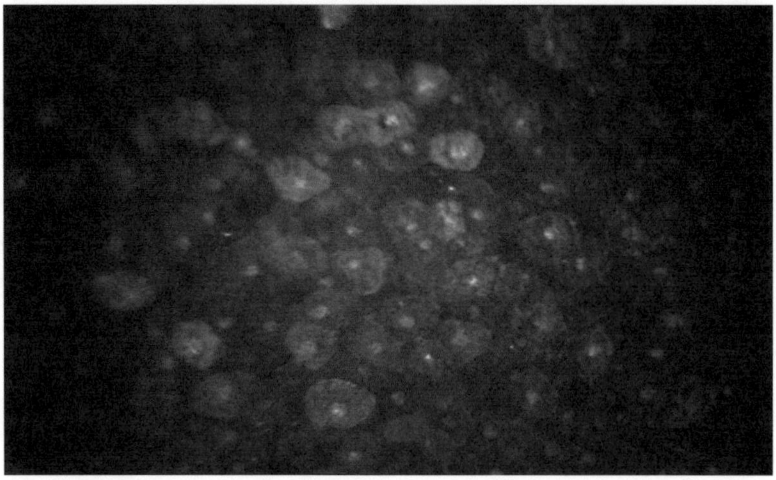

Figure 3.
Apical corneal epithelium: Layer of polygonal cells with defined edges, with a bright nucleus that stands out from the homogeneous cytoplasm. Corresponds to patient 6 months after PRK.

of surface, intermediate, and basal cells is 1: 5: 10. Basal cells have 10-15 μm in diameter and form a regular mosaic with dark cell bodies and brightness at the cell edges [14, 35] (**Figure 4**).

Langerhans cells appear as bright corpuscular particles with dendritic cell morphology and a diameter of 15 mm. Their distribution is in the form of a gradient from low numbers in the center to high cell densities in the periphery of the cornea [30, 36, 37].

The subbasal nerves are located between Bowman's membrane and the basal epithelium [38–40]. They appear as linear structures with homogeneous reflectivity, a dichotomous Y-shaped appearance, and fine H-shaped interconnecting fibers [7, 40, 41]. The membrane of Bowman is not visible by microscopy confocal. The subepithelial plexus is located between Bowman's membrane and the anterior stroma. This plexus has a diffuse, patchy distribution, apparently limited to the mid-peripheral cornea and probably absent in the central cornea [40, 42–47] (**Figure 5**).

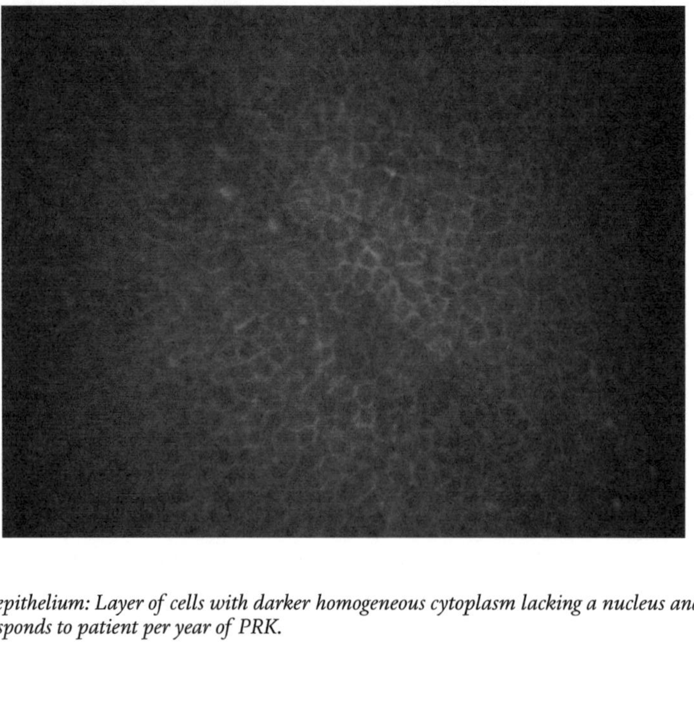

Figure 4.
Basal corneal epithelium: Layer of cells with darker homogeneous cytoplasm lacking a nucleus and defined borders. Corresponds to patient per year of PRK.

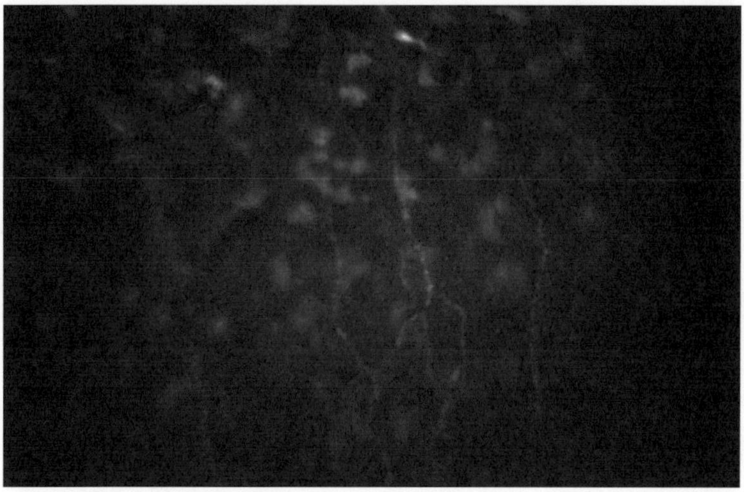

Figure 5.
Subbasal nerve plexus: Nerve fibers contrasting against the dark background, thin, bright, distributed in a parallel or oblique fashion with various interconnecting bifurcations. Corresponds to patient at LASIK year.

The stroma is seen with images of keratocyte nuclei. The cell body, keratocyte processes, and stromal collagen are not usually visible on the normal cornea. Keratocytes in the anterior stroma are well-defined images with brightness, oval, objects with varied orientation that contrast with a dark background [46, 48–51]. In the middle stroma, keratocytes have a more regular oval shape. Keratocytes in the posterior stroma appear more elongated than those in the anterior layers [22, 45, 51, 52] (**Figures 6** and 7).

Stromal nerves are located in the anterior and middle stroma, but they cannot be visualized in the posterior stroma: they appear as linear, thin, reflective structures, in various orientations, with a dichotomous pattern; internal details of the nerves are not observed [53–58].

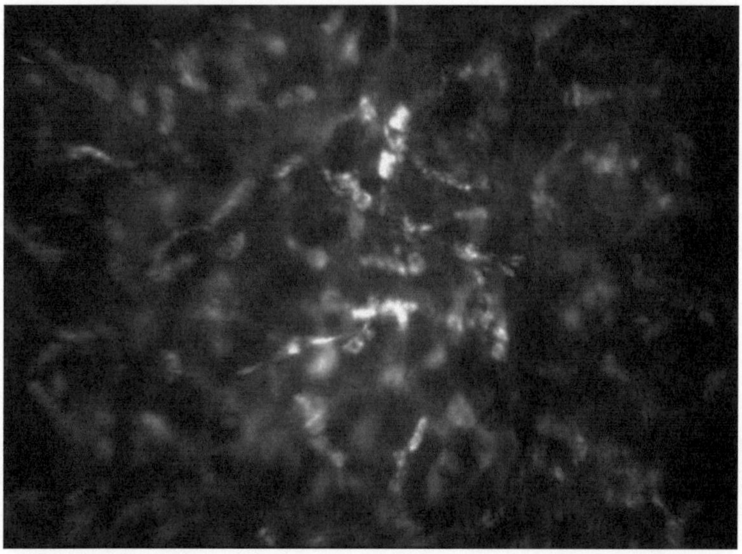

Figure 6.
Corneal stroma: Defined by the presence of bright oval bodies (keratocytes) that contrast against the dark background. Corresponds to patient 3 months after LASIK.

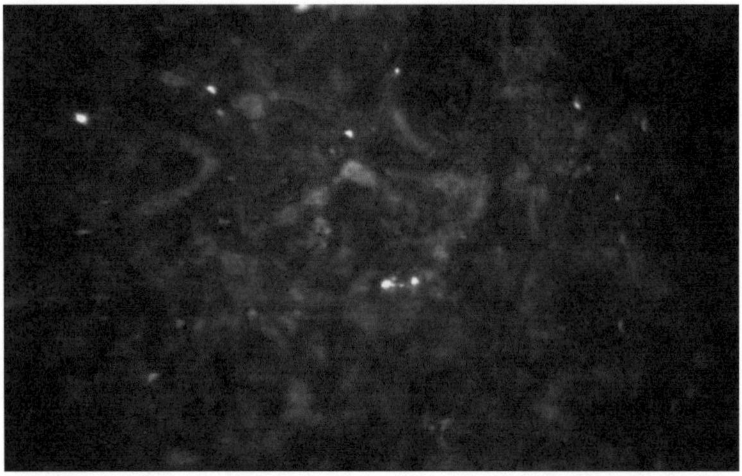

Figure 7.
Surgical interface: Presence of bright pinpoint bodies that stand out against the dark background. Corresponds to patient 1 month after LASIK.

Descemet's membrane is not visible. Endothelial cells appear as a regular hexagonal cell line exhibiting bright cell bodies with darker edges. [8, 37, 52, 59–62] (**Figure 8**).

Taking as a reference the characteristics of the normal cornea, some variables have been described after corneal refractive surgery, through confocal microscopy, such as: the thickness of the epithelium [27] and the corneal flap [16], the keratocyte cell density in different strata [50], the characteristics of corneal nerves [41], endothelial cell density, pleomorphism, polymegatism [60], corneal haze thickness [29], among other variables (**Figures 9** and **10**).

2.3 Applications of confocal microscopy of the cornea

2.3.1 Evaluation of cross linking treatment

Confocal microscopy is a diagnostic means that allows the monitoring of histological modifications that occur due to the effect of corneal crosslinking. It allows to show the recovery of the tissue in the follow-up period of the treated cases.

Among the findings, a rarefaction of keratocytes accompanied by stromal edema in the first month can be observed in the anterior-middle stroma; This can take the appearance of a trabecular network, where small elongated keratocyte nuclei can be detected corresponding to masked necrotic keratocytes and apoptotic bodies, respectively. Initial restocking generally occurs within 3 months at this depth and they regenerate almost completely within 6 months [63].

2.3.2 Corneal transplant

In confocal microscopy, we observed, in most transplanted corneas, loss of continuity of corneal nerves, absence of nerve fibers, and reduction and activation of keratocytes. When confocal microscopy findings were related to the transparency status of the graft, the absence of nerve fibers was observed in all cases of non-transparent cornea and in the vast majority of transparent corneas [64].

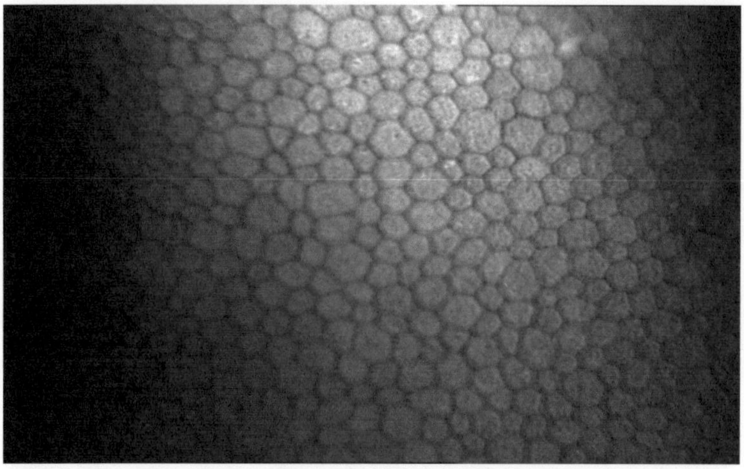

Figure 8.
Corneal endothelium: Hexagonal cells with defined edges, anucleated, with homogeneous cytoplasm. Corresponds to patient per year of PRK.

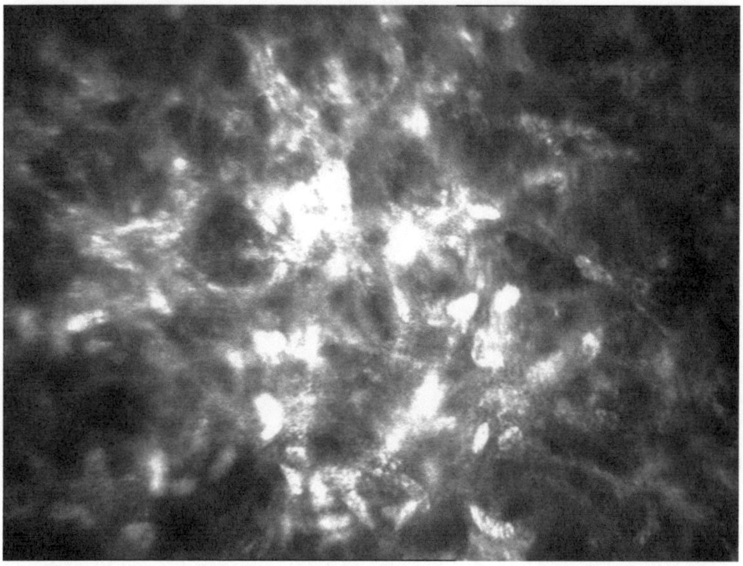

Figure 9.
Corneal haze, the keratocyte limits cannot be defined, with greater brightness than the rest of the stromal images. Corresponds to patient 3 months after PRK.

2.3.3 Corneal dystrophies

Sometimes it is difficult to make the differential diagnosis between different types of corneal dystrophies using only slit lamp biomicroscopy, hence the importance of confocal microscopy in the study of dystrophies.

For example, in a patient with a diagnosis of basement membrane dystrophy, reduplication of the basement membrane is observed, in Meesmann's dystrophies hyporeflectic areas in the basal layer of the epithelium, mostly circular, oval or drop-shaped, with a range of 48 and 145 μm in diameter [65].

In Thiel-Behnke dystrophy, deposits are observed in the basal layer of the corneal epithelium of homogeneous reflectivity with curved filaments accompanied

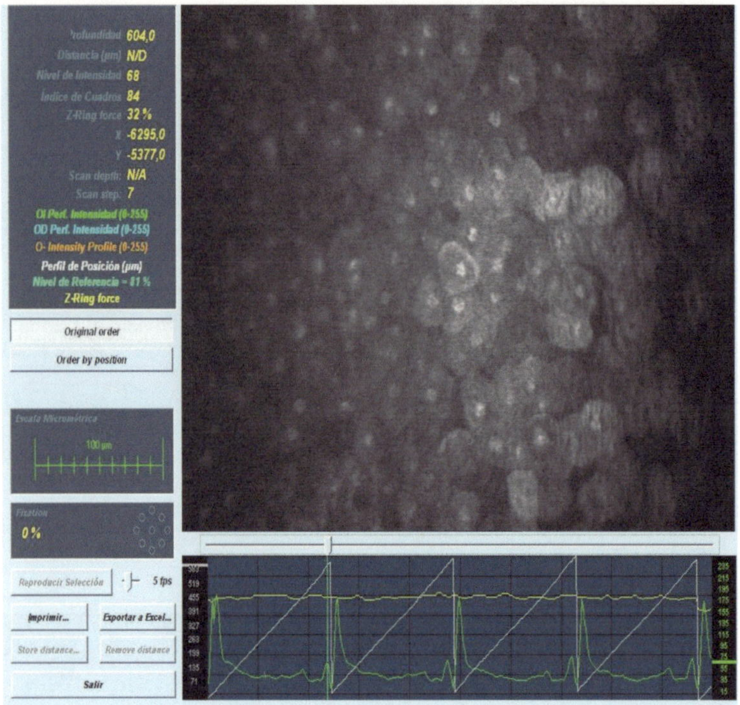

Figure 10.
Pachymetry measurement. Pachymetry is the value illustrated as depth in the upper left of the CMTF curve image. The example is 6 months after LASIK.

by dark shadows. Meanwhile, in corneas with Reis-Bücklers dystrophy, in the same layer, deposits with extremely high reflectivity are observed from small granular materials [65].

In granular dystrophy by confocal microscopy, the superficial epithelium is normal in appearance, while in the basal epithelium, highly reflective deposits are observed without defined borders. High reflectivity deposits are also observed in the superficial stroma. At Bowman's membrane level, sub-basal nerves with a raised fundus can be seen [65].

In keratoconus, the epithelium shows the following characteristics: elongated, spindle-shaped surface cells, larger and irregularly spaced nuclei of wing cells, and flattened basal cells. Images obtained using confocal microscopy reveal the disruption of Bowman's layer and the occasional presence of epithelial cells and stromal keratocytes [65].

2.3.4 Corneal refractive surgery

The confocal microscope has been widely used in the study of patients after refractive procedures. Modifications have been described at the level of different sublayers of the cornea, showing high reliability and reproducibility for these purposes [66–69].

Confocal microscopy allows the visualization of the stromal flap in LASIK, the analysis of its thickness and regularity, the density of corneal cells by stromal sublayers, the exact obtaining of the residual corneal bed, the study of the modifications of the subbasal nervous plexus and the nerves, stromal cells, as well as their recovery after this surgery. It allows the study of corneal haze in PRK, its evolution and response to treatment [66–69] (**Figures 11–19**).

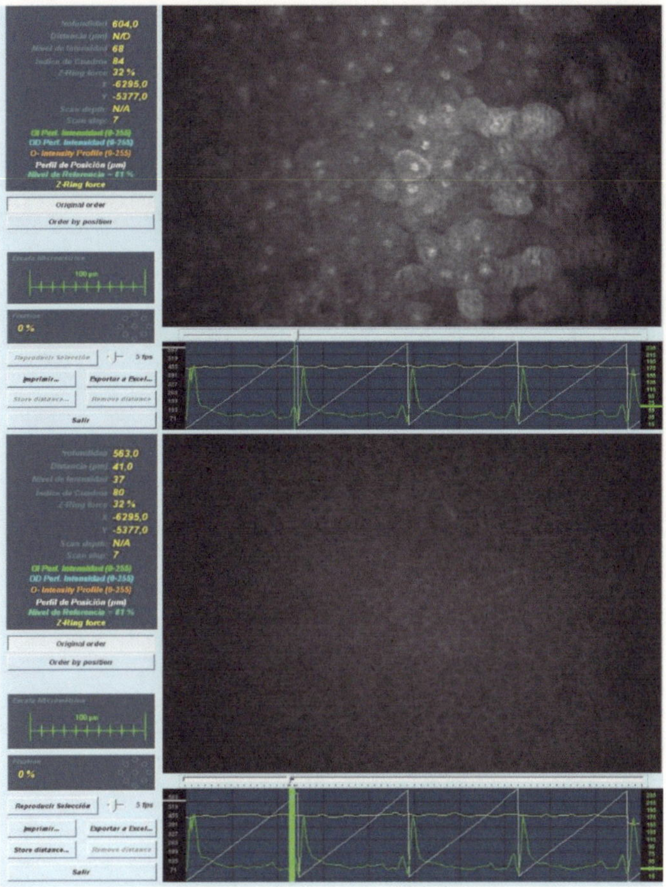

Figure 11.
Measurement of epithelial thickness. The most anterior apical corneal epithelium image is selected by CMTF curve (upper image) and the cursor is moved to the last basal corneal epithelium image. (lower image) epithelial thickness is the value illustrated as distance (µm) = 41 in the upper left of the lower image. The example is 6 months after LASIK.

2.3.5 Infectious keratitis

Confocal microscopy is emerging as an important technique in the early diagnosis of various corneal entities. It is capable of providing magnifications close to 200x-500x, providing images with high detail and contrast levels, even in opacified corneas. Its non-invasive nature makes it an especially useful technique in the diagnosis of infectious keratitis caused by Acanthamoeba. In addition, it allows repeated examinations, which helps the diagnosis, monitoring and taking therapeutic attitudes. Typical lesions correspond to amoebic cyst or trophozoite (hyperreflective lesions surrounded by a double wall and a peripheral halo), and radial keratoneuritis (linear hyperreflective thickening). Therefore, when faced with a patient who develops nonspecific manifestations of infectious keratitis, the possibility of performing this test should not be forgotten, in conjunction with histological studies, since it gives us the possibility of an early diagnosis and a better prognosis [70].

2.3.6 Patients with retinal surgeries

We can inspect corneal morphology at the cellular level in patients with emulsified silicone oil in the anterior chamber, which contributes to detecting

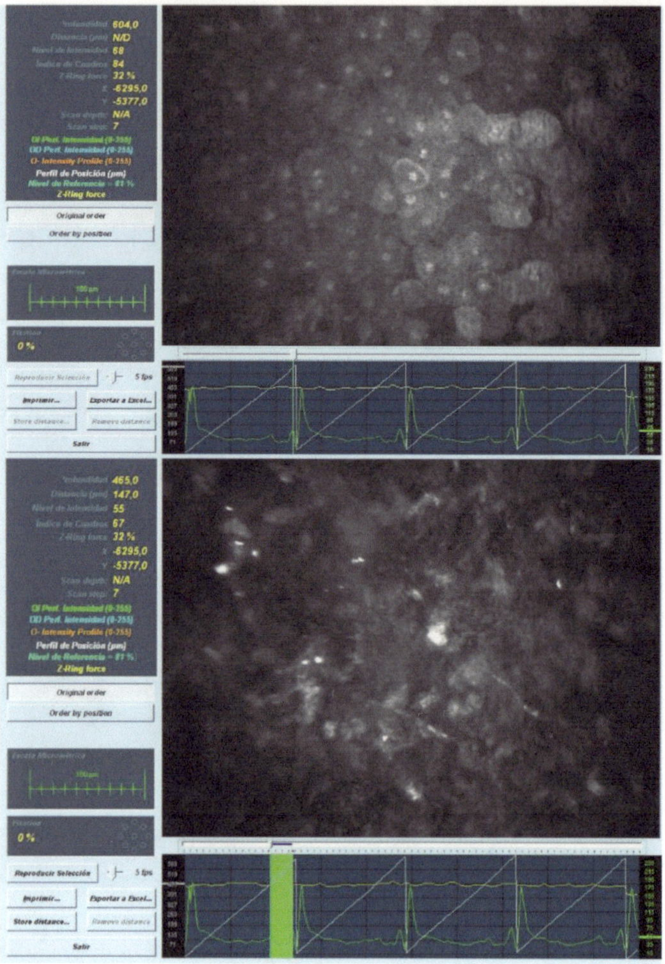

Figure 12.
Flap thickness measurement. The first apical corneal epithelium image (upper image) is selected on the CMTF curve and the cursor is moved to the first surgical interface image (lower image). The thickness of the flap is the value illustrated as distance (μm) = 147 in the upper left of the lower image. The example is 6 months after LASIK.

early histological changes, both morphological and morphometric that guide us towards a behavior to avoid subsequent tissue damage.

Images obtained through confocal microscopy show different degrees of polymegatism and pleomorphism, hyperreflectivity determined by deposits of emulsified silicone oil on the corneal endothelium that are seen as bright or elongated stippling, activation of keratocytes in the stroma with loss of the matrix extracellular by contact with oil, multidots lesions and in some cases folds of the descemet [71].

2.3.7 Diabetic patients

Diabetes mellitus is the most common endocrine disorder in ophthalmic practice, and disorders of the anterior segment are less frequently described than those of the retina, although they are present in many patients. This disease affects the biomechanics of the corneal epithelium and endothelium, causes a significant effect on the morphology, metabolism and clinical and physiological aspects of the cornea. The metabolic disorders typical of diabetics constitute an important factor in the appearance of diabetic neuropathy and other subsequent pathologies.

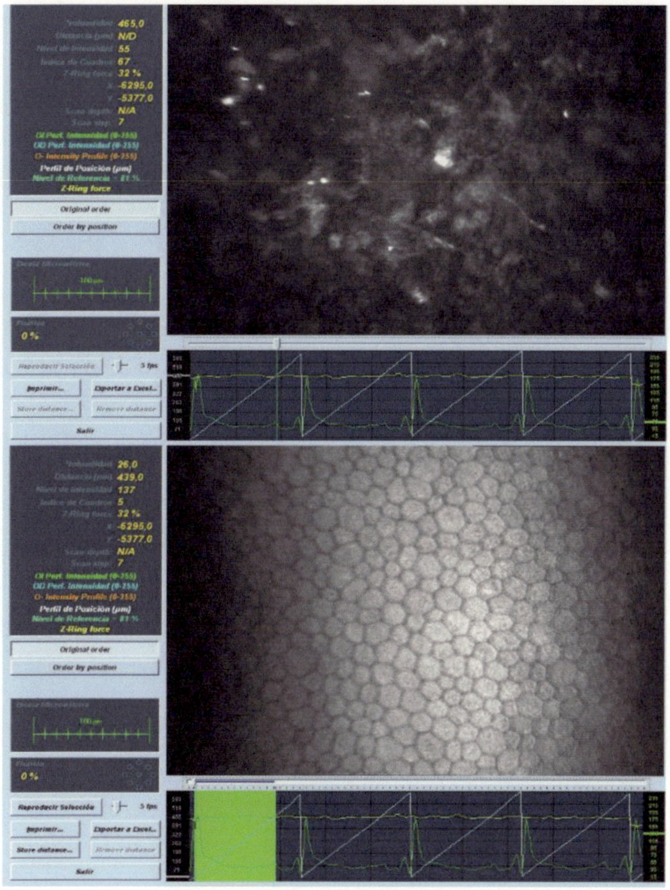

Figure 13.
Measurement of residual stromal bed (3 months after LASIK). Using the CMTF curve, the last surgical interface image (upper image) is selected and the cursor is moved to the last image of corneal endothelium (lower image). The residual stromal bed thickness is the value illustrated as distance (µm) = 439.0 in the upper left of the lower image. The example is 3 months after LASIK.

In confocal microscopy, a decrease in the density of the sub-basal nerve plexus can be observed with an increase in its thickness and tortuosity, a decrease in the density of the nerve fibers of the sub-basal nerve plexus, as well as the association of certain changes morphological of these as: fewer branches, shorter lengths, as well as increased tortuosity and presence of edema.

Greater total corneal thickness and layers are observed, the basement membrane is visible in diabetic patients. There is a decrease in the sub-basal nervous plexus with vertical disposition and an increase in the tortuosity of the nerve fibers [72].

2.3.8 Filtering bull in glaucoma

The confocal scanning laser microscope with the Rostock corneal module is a revolutionary element in the monitoring of glaucoma operated patients. The presence of encapsulated stromal cysts surrounded by a hyperreflective line that defines them and separates them from the rest of the structures (capsule) can be evaluated. Besides the visualization of thick conjunctival vessels that describe curves in their course (tortuous); On the other hand, the size of the filtering bullet is evaluable, through the measurement of the dimensions of the bullet in its largest diameter [73].

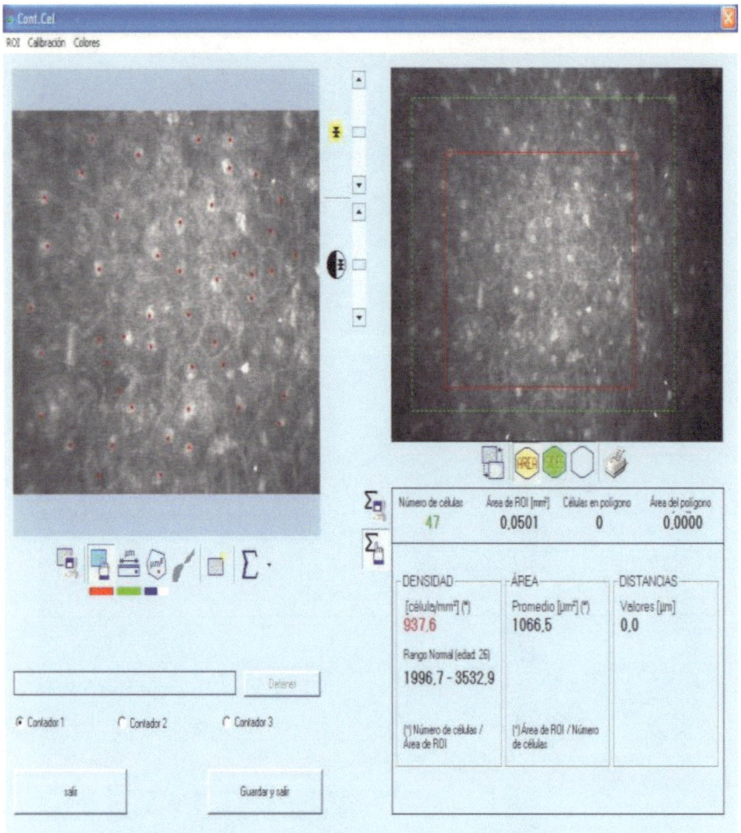

Figure 14.
Calculation of the cell density of the apical epithelium. After selecting the image and the ROI area (0.0500 mm^2), the cells are marked in the upper left image and the density value is obtained through the software, in this case 937.6 cells/mm^2. The example corresponds to 6 months after PRK).

2.4 Method of use of the corneal confocal microscope. Calculations and images obtained

The NIDEK ConfoScan four confocal microscope is shown for obtaining and studying in vivo images of corneal tissue. The Z ring must be attached for fixation of the eyeball with the 40x lens. It is programmed in automatic scanning mode, with central fixation, image acquisition speed of 25 images per second, 500x magnification, 0.6 µm/pixel lateral resolution, with 350 images per scan, 1.98 mm working distance.

Anesthetic eye drops and subsequently Viscotears (gel) are instilled as a coupling medium between the cornea and the Z ring. The lens is advanced until the ring is contacted with the coupling substance. The objective lens is aligned with the center of the cornea until the first images of corneal epithelium are observed. The digital images obtained are captured automatically and recorded on a computer for later analysis. Before and after each examination, the objective lens is cleaned with isopropyl alcohol.

Each image obtained is separated from the adjacent image by four microns, 25 µm depth of field, intensity level 0 to 255, Z-ring pressure 20%. All shots belong to the central four mm of the cornea.

The necessary examinations are performed in each patient until obtaining, by full-focus quantitative confocal microscopy (CMTF curve), scans and images of maximum stability in terms of pressure applied by the Z ring with variations of less than 10%, represented by the yellow curve. The selected images should not be modified in brightness and contrast, the analysis is carried out with the NAVIS software.

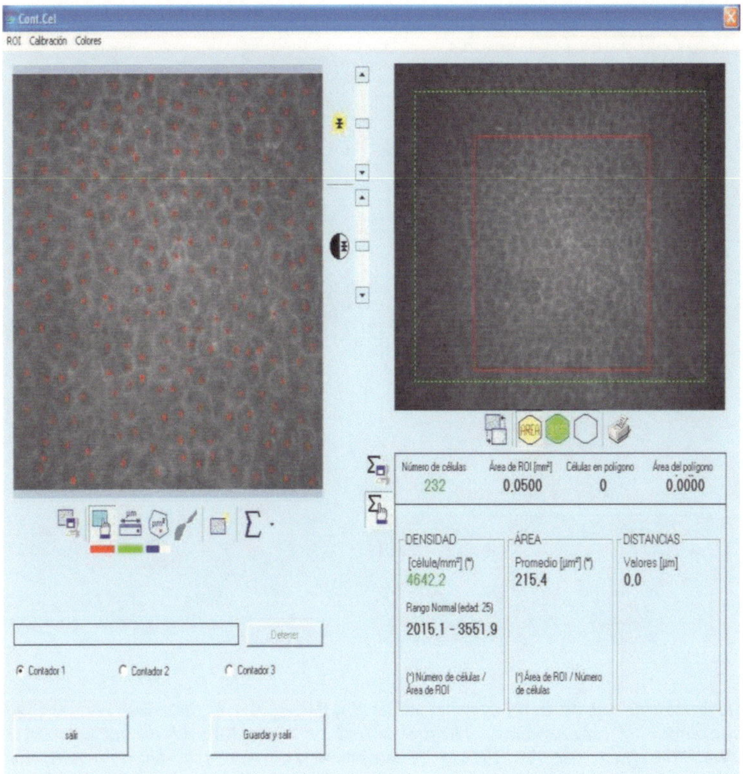

Figure 15.
Calculation of basal epithelium cell density. After selecting the image and the ROI area (0.0500 mm²), the cells are marked in the upper left image and the density value is obtained through the software, in this case 4642 cells/mm². Example corresponds to 1 year after PRK).

Steps to follow in microscopy. A: Z ring for fixation of the eyeball. B: 40X lens. C: Coupling of A and B. D: The lens was advanced until contacting the ring with the coupling substance for examination.

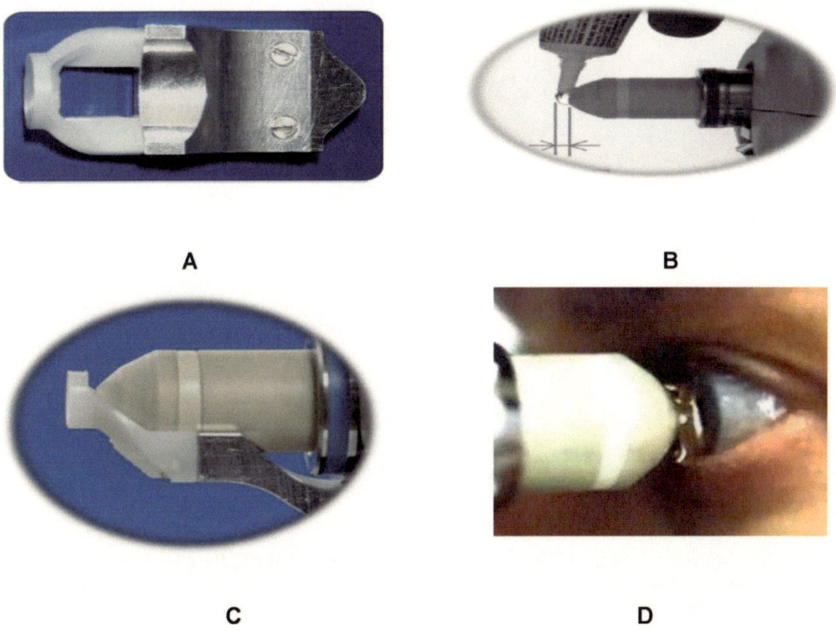

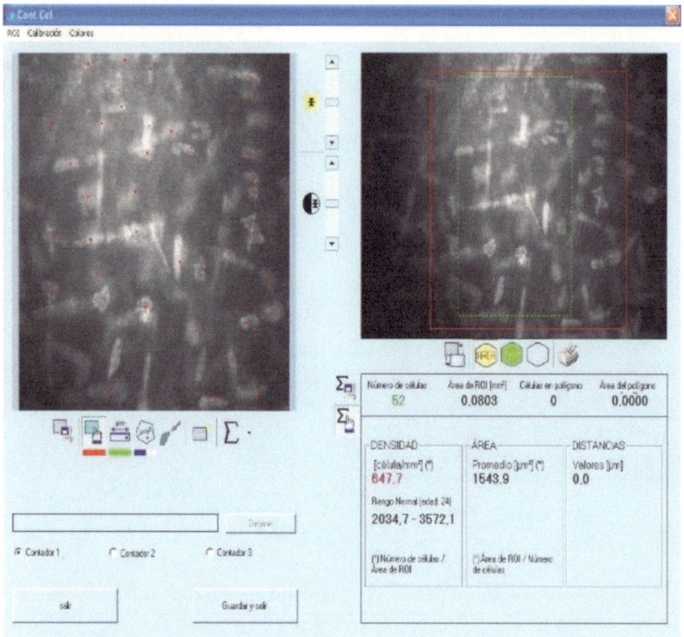

Figure 16.
Calculation of keratocyte density. In the upper right portion the selection of the area is observed, in the upper left portion the marking of each keratocyte. The first density quotient obtained is the one with red letters. This value is divided by the effective depth of field of the equipment: 25 to obtain the density in cells/mm³.

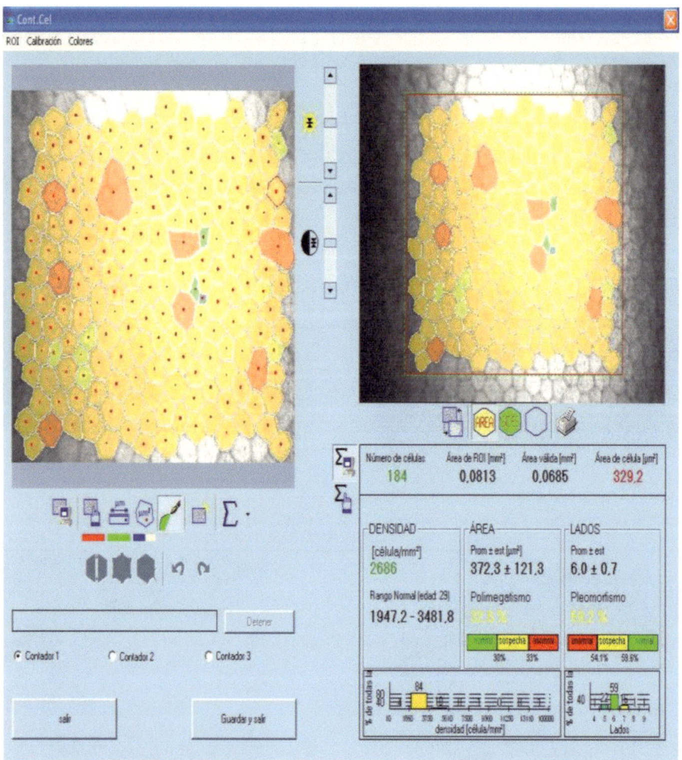

Figure 17.
Calculation of endothelial variables. In the upper right portion the selection of the area is observed, in the upper left portion the automatic marking of the cells. In the lower portion, the values obtained for endothelial cell density, pleomorphism and polymegatism are observed.

DOI: http://dx.doi.org/10.5772/intechopen.96272

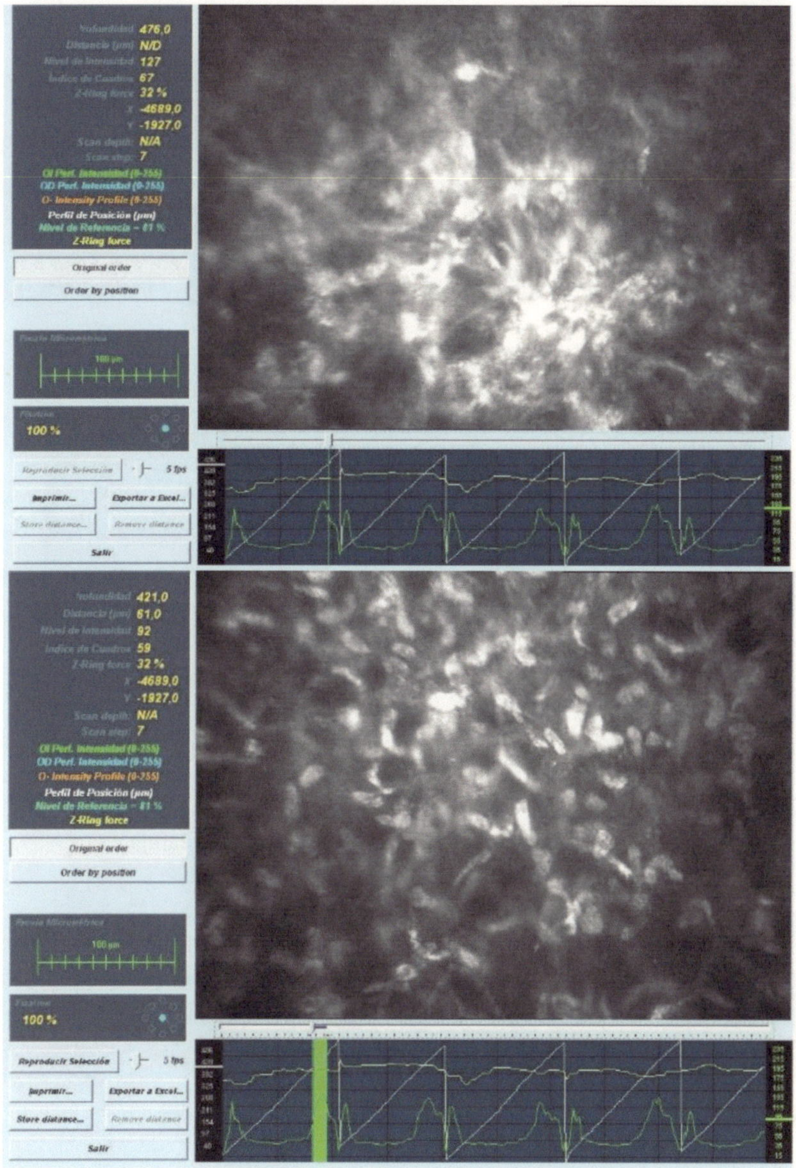

Figure 18.
Measurement of corneal haze, after PRK. In this case, 3 months after PRK, the upper image shows a CMTF curve, taking the first image of corneal haze, then the cursor is moved to the last image of corneal haze shown in the lower figure, where the parameter called distance = 61 μm.

The lower right part shows the quality of the shot given by the constancy of the yellow line and the uniformity of the white line. The green line corresponds to the reflectivity in the form of peaks. An image of corneal epithelium belonging to the first image of the 4 existing ones is shown.

Full focus quantitative confocal microscopy (CMTF), where the selected image is seen in the upper right: Apical epithelium one year after LASIK.

The top left shows the parameters of depth, distance, intensity level, pressure of the Z ring, among others. The lower right part shows the quality of the shot given by the constancy of the yellow line and the uniformity of the white line. The green line corresponds to the reflectivity in the form of peaks. An image of corneal epithelium belonging to the first image of the 4 existing ones is shown.

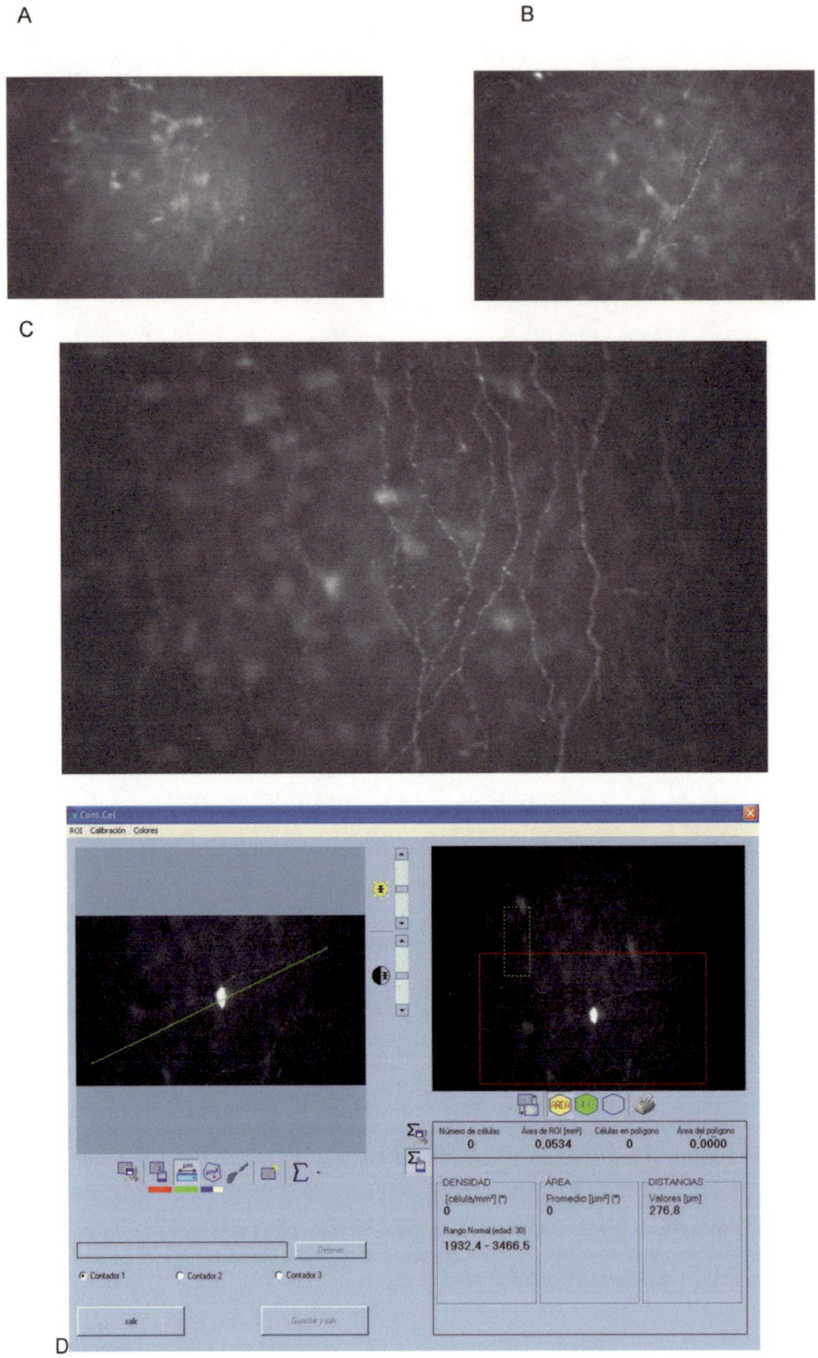

Figure 19.
Subbasal nerve plexus. (A) Short nerve, less than 200 µm in length. (B) Long nerve (greater than 200 µm without interconnections). (C) Nerves long with interconnections. (D) Measurement of the nerve.

3. Conclusions

The corneal study by confocal microscopy allows the differentiation of epithelium sublayers, subbasal nerve plexus, keratocytes, stromal nerves, and corneal endothelium cells.

Its usefulness has been demonstrated in the study of patients with corneal dystrophies, keratoconus, infectious keratitis, corneal refractive surgery, it has also shown usefulness in the study of patients with corneal transplantation, corneal crosslinking, diabetics, vitrectomized, as well as the study of the filtering bulla in glaucoma.

It is necessary to continue improving the methods of calculation and identification of structures by cornea confocal microscopy, in order to obtain better images and analyzes that contribute to more accurate diagnoses and broaden the spectrum utility of this novel technology.

Conflict of interest

I confirm there are no conflicts of interest.

Author details

Eduardo Rojas Alvarez[1,2]

1 Faculty of Medical Sciences, University of Cuenca, Ecuador

2 Exilaser Ophthalmology Center, Ecuador

*Address all correspondence to: drerojasalvarez@gmail.com

References

[1] Martínez R, Iviricu R, Correa O, Blanco A, Acosta L. Frecuencia de ametropías diagnosticadas en consulta de cirugía refractiva. Rev CIGET Pinar del Río. 2008;10(3).

[2] Tomita M, Kanamori T, Waring GO, Yukawa S, Yamamoto T, Sekiya K, et al. Simultaneous corneal inlay implantation and laser in situ keratomileusis for presbyopia in patients with hyperopia, myopia, or emmetropia: Six- month results. J Cataract & Refract Surg. 2012;38(3):495-506.

[3] Christopoulos V, Kagemann L, Wollstein G, Ishikawa H, Gabriele M, Wojtkowski M, et al. In vivo corneal high-speed, ultra–high-resolution optical coherence tomography. Arch Ophthalmol. 2007;125(8):1027-1035.

[4] Alió JL. Laser refractive surgery: have we arrived? Br J Ophthalmol. 2012;96(9):1159.

[5] Winkler C, Khoramnia R, Salgado J, Wullner C, Donitzky C, Mathias M, et al. First clinical results with a new 200 kHz femtosecond laser system. Br J Ophthalmol. 2012;96(6):788-792.

[6] Miri A, Alomar T, Nubile M, Al-Agaba M, Lanzini M, Fares U, et al. In vivo confocal microscopic findings in patients with limbal stem cell deficiency. Br J Ophthalmol. 2012;96(4):523-529.

[7] Zhivov A, Guthoff RF, Stachs O. In vivo confocal microscopy of the ocular surface: from bench to bedside and back again. Br J Ophthalmol. 2010;94(12):1557-1558.

[8] Erie JC, McLaren JW, Patel SV. Confocal microscopy in ophthalmology. Am J Ophthalmol. 2009;148(5):639-634.

[9] Miri A, Al-Agaba M, Muneer A, Fares U, Said D, Faraj LA, et al. In vivo confocal microscopic features of normal limbus. Br J Ophthalmol. 2012;96(4):530-536.

[10] Tavakoli M, Hossain P, Malik RA. Clinical applications of corneal confocal microscopy. Clinical Ophathalmology. 2008;2(2):435-445.

[11] Zhivov A, Stachs O, Stave J, Guthoff RF. In vivo three-dimensional confocal laser scanning microscopy of corneal surface and epithelium. Br J Ophthalmol. 2009;93(5):667-672.

[12] Villani E, Galimberti D, Viola F, Ratiglia R. In vivo confocal microscopy of the ocular surface. Am J Ophthalmol. 2010;149(4):689-690.

[13] Kobayashi A, Mawatari Y, Yokogawa H, Sugiyama K. In vivo laser confocal microscopy after descemet stripping with automated endothelial keratoplasty. Am J Ophthalmol. 2008;145(6):977-985.

[14] Guthoff RF, Zhivov A, Stachs O. In vivo confocal microscopy, an inner vision of the cornea - a major review. Clin Experiment Ophthalmol. 2009;37(1):100-117.

[15] Petroll WM, Cavanagh HD. Remote-Controlled scanning and automated confocal microscopy through-focusing using a modified HRT Rostock Corneal Module. Eye Contact Lens. 2009;35(6):302-308.

[16] Javaloy J, Vidal MT, Ruiz JM, Alió JL. Microscopía confocal de la córnea en la cirugía foforrefractiva. Arch Soc Esp Oftalmol. 2005;80(9):497-509.

[17] Ramírez M, Martínez Y, Naranjo R. Hallazgos mediante microscopía confocal en pacientes postoperados de LASIK tratados con antiinflamatorios no esteroideos (AINES). Rev Mex Oftalmol. 2008;82(6):349-351.

[18] Nubile M, Mastropasqua L. In vivo confocal microscopy of the ocular surface: where are we now? Br J Ophthalmol 2009;93(7):850-852.

[19] Reynolds A, Moore JE, Naroo SA, Moore T, Shah S. Excimer laser surface ablation - a review. Clin & Experiment Ophthalmol. 2010;38(2):168-182.

[20] Reinstein DZ, Threlfall WB, Cook R, Cremonesi E, Sutton H, Archer T, et al. Short term LASIK outcomes using the Technolas 217C excimer laser and Hansatome microkeratome in 46 708 eyes treated between 1998 and 2001. Br J Ophthalmol. 2012; 96(9):1173-1179.

[21] Mastropasqua L, Nubile M, Lanzini M, Carpineto P, Ciancaglini M, Pannellini T, et al. Epithelial dendritic cell distribution in normal and inflamed human cornea: in vivo confocal microscopy study. Am J Ophthalmol. 2006;142(5):736-744.

[22] Nishida T. The cornea: stasis and dynamics. Nihon Ganka Gakkai Zasshi.2008;112(3):179-212.

[23] Sherwin T. Corneal epithelial homeostasis. Ophthalmology. 2010;117:190-191.

[24] Reichard M, Hovakimyan M, Wree A, Meyer A, Nolte I, Junghans C. Comparative in vivo confocal microscopical study of the cornea anatomy of different laboratory animals. Curr Eye Res. 2010;35(12):1072-1080.

[25] DelMonte DW, Kim T. Anatomy and physiology of the cornea. J Cataract Refract Surg. 2011;37(3):588-598.

[26] Mootha V, Dawson D, Kumar A, Gleiser J, Qualls C, Albert DM. Slitlamp, specular, and light microscopic findings of human donor corneas after laser-assisted in situ keratomileusis. Arch Ophthalmol. 2004;122(5):686-692.

[27] Ivarsen A, Fledelius W, Hjortdal J. Three-year changes in epithelial and stromal thickness after PRK or LASIK for high myopia. Invest. Ophthalmol. Vis. Sci. 2009;50(5):2061-2066.

[28] Dvorscak L, Marfurt C. Age-related changes in rat corneal epithelial nerve density. Invest Ophthalmol Vis Sci. 2008;49(3):910-916.

[29] Pérez-Gómez I, Efron N. Change to corneal morphology after refractive surgery (myopic in situ keratomileusis) as viewed with a confocal microscope. Optom Vis Sci. 2003;80(10):690-697.

[30] Cruzat A, Zheng L, Hamrah P. In vivo confocal microscopy study of epithelial dendritic cells and subbasal nerve plexus in infectious keratitis. 26th Biennial Cornea Conference Abstracts 2009;Boston, MA.

[31] Deng SX, Seipal KD, Tang Q, Aldave AJ, Lee O, Yu F. Characterization of limbal stem cell deficiency by in vivo laser scanning confocal microscopy: a microstructural approach. Arch Ophthalmol. 2012;130(4):440-445.

[32] Masters BR, Böhnke M. Three-dimensional confocal microscopy of the living human eye. Annu Rev Biomed Eng. 2002;4:69-91.

[33] Patel DV, Sherwin T, McGhee CH. Laser scanning in vivo confocal microscopy of the normal human corneoscleral limbus. Invest. Ophthalmol. Vis. Sci. 2006;47(7):2823-2827.

[34] Barbaro V, Ferrari S, Fasolo A, Pedrotti E, Marchini G, Sbabo A, et al. Evaluation of ocular surface disorders: a new diagnostic tool based on impression cytology and confocal laser scanning microscopy. Br J Ophthalmol 2010;94(7):926-932.

[35] Ehlers N, Heegaard S, Hjortdal J, Ivarsen A, Nielsen K, Prause JU.

Morphological evaluation of normal human corneal epithelium. Acta Ophthalmology. 2010;88(8):858-861.

[36] Ivarsen A, Laurberg T, Møller-Pedersen T. Characterisation of corneal fibrotic wound repair at the LASIK flap margin. Br J Ophthalmol. 2003;87(10):1272-1278.

[37] Kobayashi A. In vivo laser confocal microscopic analysis of the interface between Bowman's layer and the stroma of the cornea. Nihon Ganka Gakkai Zasshi. 2008;112:947-952.

[38] Scarpa F, Zheng X, Ohashi Y, Ruggeri A. Automatic evaluation of corneal nerve tortuosity in images from in vivo confocal microscopy. Invest. Ophthalmol. Vis. Sci. 2011;52(9):6404-6408.

[39] Zhivov A, Blum M, Guthoff R, Stachs O. Real-time mapping of the subepithelial nerve plexus by in vivo confocal laser scanning microscopy. Br J Ophthalmol. 2010;94(9):1133-1135.

[40] Allgeier S, Zhivov A, Eberle F, Koehler B, Maier S, Bretthauer G, et al. Image reconstruction of the subbasal nerve plexus within vivo confocal microscopy. Invest. Ophthalmol. Vis. Sci. 2011;52(9):5022-5028.

[41] Patel SV, McLaren JW, Kittleson KM, Bourne WM. Subbasal nerve density and corneal sensitivity after laser in situ keratomileusis femtosecond laser vs mechanical microkeratome. Arch Ophthalmol. 2010;128(11):1413-1419.

[42] Erie EA, McLaren JW, Kittleson KM, Patel SV, Erie JC, Bourne W. Corneal subbasal nerve density: A comparison of two confocal microscopes. Eye Contact Lens. 2008;34(6):322-325.

[43] Cruzat A, Pavan-Langston D, Hamrah P. In vivo confocal microscopy of corneal nerves: analysis and clinical correlation. Semin Ophthalmol. 2010;25(5):171-177.

[44] Grupcheva CN, Wong T, Riley AF, McGhee CN. Assessing the sub-basal nerve plexus of the living healthy human cornea by in vivo confocal microscopy. Clin Experiment Ophthalmol. 2002;30(3):187-190.

[45] Esquenazi S, He J, Li N, Bazan NG, Esquenazi I, Bazan HE. Comparative in vivo high-resolution confocal microscopy of corneal epithelium, sub- basal nerves and stromal cells in mice with and without dry eye after photorefractive keratectomy. Clin Experiment Ophthalmol. 2007;35(6):545-

[46] Pacheco C, Baca O, Velasco R. Reinervación corneal y dinámica de queratocitos posterior a queratoplastía penetrante. Reporte de casos. Rev Mex Oftalmol. 2008;82(4):263-266.

[47] Patel DV, McGhee CN. In vivo laser scanning confocal microscopy confirms that the human corneal sub-basal nerve plexus is a highly dynamic structure. Invest Ophthalmol Vis Sci. 2008;49(8):3409-3412.

[48] Mimura T, Amano S, Yokoo S, Uchida S, Usui T, Yamagami S. Isolation and distribution of rabbit keratocyte precursors. Mol Vis. 2008;14:197-203.

[49] Weaving L, Mihelec M, Storen R, Sosic D, Grigg JR, Patrick PL, et al. Twist2: Role in corneal stromal keratocyte proliferation and corneal thickness. Invest. Ophthalmol. Vis. Sci. 2010;51(11):5561-5570.

[50] Javadi M, Mozhgan K, Manijeh M, Mehdi Y, Hosein R, Atefeh J, et al. Comparison of keratocyte density between keratoconus, post-laser in situ keratomileusis keratectasia, and uncomplicated post-laser in situ keratomileusis cases. A confocal scan study. Cornea. 2009;28(7):774-779.

[51] Argento C, Croxatt JO. Evaluación de la celularidad estromal corneal mediante microscopía confocal en LASEK con Mitomicina. Oftalmol Clin Exp. 2007;35(1):14-20.

[52] Niederer RL, McGhee CN. Clinical in vivo confocal microscopy of the human cornea in health and disease. Prog Retin Eye Res. 2010;29(1):30.

[53] Zhao Ch, Lu S, Tajouri N, Dosso A, Safran A. In vivo confocal laser scanning microscopy of corneal nerves in leprosy. Arch Ophthalmol. 2008;126(2):282-284.

[54] Marfurt CF, Deek S, Dvorscak L. Anatomy of the human corneal innervation. Exp Eye Res. 2010;90:478-492.

[55] Al-Faky Y, Bosley T, Turki T, Salih M, Abu-Amero K, Alsuhaibani A. Prominent corneal nerves: a novel sign of lipoid proteinosis. Br J Ophthalmol. 2012;96(7):935-940.

[56] Al-Aqaba MA, Fares U, Suleman H, Lowe J, Dua HS. Architecture and distribution of human corneal nerves. Br J Ophthalmol. 2010;94(6):784-789.

[57] Karagianni N, Fukuoka S. Analysis of corneal nerve regeneration following deep vs. superficial injury. ARVO Meeting Abstracts. 2010;51:392.

[58] Jiucheng H, Bazan N, Bazan H. Mapping the entire human corneal nerve architecture. Exp Eye Res. 2010;91(4):513-523.

[59] Vanathi M, Tandon R, Sharma N, Titiyal JS, Pandey RM, Vajpayee RB. In-vivo slit scanning confocal microscopy of normal corneas in Indian eyes. Indian J Ophthalmol. 2003;51(3):225-230.

[60] Patel SV, Bourne W. Corneal endothelial cell loss 9 years after excimer laser keratorefractive surgery. Arch Ophthalmol. 2009;127(11):1423-1427.

[61] Lagali N, Dellby A, Fagerholm P. In vivo confocal microscopy of the cornea in Darier-White disease. Arch Ophthalmol. 2009;127(6):816-818.

[62] Lautebach S, Funk J, Reinhard T, Pache M. Steroid glaucoma after laser in situ keratomileusis. Klin Monatsbl Augenheilkd. 2007; 224(5):438-440.

[63] Jareño Ochoa M, Pérez Parra Z, Fernández García K, Castillo Pérez A, Escalona Leyva E, Ruíz Rodríguez Y. Changes in the cell structure of patients with keratoconus under cross-linking treatment by using confocal microscopy. Rev Cubana Ophthalmology. 2012; 25 (2).

[64] Pérez Parra Z, Padilla González C, Jareño Ochoa M, Gómez Castillo Z, Guerra Almaguer M, Sibila González M. Corneal changes after penetrating optical keratoplasty. Rev Cubana Ophthalmology. 2017; 30 (1).

[65] González–Sotero J, Casanueva-Cabeza HC, Alberro-Hernández M, Rojas-Alvarez E. Microscopía confocal en las distrofias corneales. ARCH. OFTAL. B. AIRES; vol 82 n° 1; pág 33-39; 2011.

[66] Rojas Alvarez E, González Sotero J. Sequential confocal microscopy of corneal nerve regeneration in myopia surgery by PRK. Rev Mex Oftalmol . 2018; 92 (3).

[67] Rojas-Alvarez E, González-Sotero J. Quantitative confocal microscopy of corneal haze and correlation with the ametropy to be treated, in surface refractive surgery. Rev Mex Oftalmol 2016;90:159-166.

[68] Rojas-Alvarez E, González-Sotero J. Tamargo Barbeíto T. Corneal morphometric predictive models from ametropia to excimer laser treatment. Arch Soc Esp Oftalmol 2015;90:312-323.

[69] Rojas-Alvarez E, González-Sotero J (2013). LASIK vs. LASEK: in vivo

corneal morphometrical perspective. Rev Mex Oftalmol 2013; 87(3): 145-157. 2013.

[70] Álvarez Marín J, Rodríguez Gil R, Alfonso Rodríguez A, Abreu Reyes p. Application of confocal microscopy in the diagnosis of Acanthamoeba keratitis. Archivos de la Sociedad Canaria de Oftalmología. 2011; 22: 14-19.

[71] Veitía Rovirosa ZN, García Ramos L, Bauza Fortunato Y, Pérez Candelaria EC, Rodríguez Suárez B, Méndez Duque de Estrada AM. Use of the confocal microscopy in patients vitrectomized with silicone oil in their anterior chamber. Rev Cubana Ophthalmology. 2014; 27 (2).

[72] Gutiérrez Castillo M, Castillo Pérez AC, Ramos López M, Pérez Parra Z, Ramos Pereira Y, Barroso Lorenzo R. Confocal microscopy of the cornea in diabetic patients. ReV Cubana de Ophthalmology. 2020;33(1)e692.

[73] Ferrer Guerra MT, Díaz Águila Y, Fernández Argones L, Piloto Díaz I, Domínguez Randulfe M, Obret Mendive I. Confocal laser scanning microscopy and its association to the morphology of the filtering bleb. Rev Cubana Ophthalmology. 2012; 25 (2).

Section 3

Radiation Safety and Stroke Detection

Chapter 5

Occupational Health and Radiation Safety of Radiography Workers

Hasna Albander

Abstract

Medical imaging is the identification or study procedure for obtaining medical images of body parts. Millions of imaging procedures take place worldwide each week. Radiation protection is intended to prevent the ionizing radiation exposure from having harmful effects. Exposure may result from a source of radiation outside the human body, or from ingestion of radioactive pollution from internal irradiation. This chapter presents Occupational Health and Radiation Safety of Radiography workers in the medical imaging field. This chapter also summarizes how current employment health status and knowledge gaps can be illustrated in some key and critical occupational issues as well as diseases such as radiation, nosocomial and occupational infections.

Keywords: occupational, health, radiation safety, radiography, workers

1. Introduction

Occupation Safety and Health (OSH) is a multidisciplinary sector dedicated to worker safety and welfare [1, 2]. The goal of this organization is to promote a safe, healthy work environment through a workplace health and safety program. Common law enforces employers to take proper care of employee safety [3, 4]. The legal system can also impose other general functions, set specific tasks, and setup government regulatory bodies. [5] OSH can also protect coworkers, families, workers, employers, and many others who affected by the working environment. As hospitals focus on disease transmission, they are also places for the sick. Everyone with a health problem is more vulnerable to infection, so controlling infection is crucial in patient care [6, 7]. As a medical team member, the infection control policy considers as one of radiography worker's professional duties. This promotes patient safety, radiographers and other health team members. The emergence of new diseases, their return, and the development of hospital-acquired multi-drug - resistant infections make it even more important to implement such policies and to play a role in preventing spread of infection [8]. Microorganisms are living organisms that are too small to see. Including bacteria, viruses, protozoa, fungi, and prions. Most microorganisms are not infectious or disease-free and essential to our well-being. Normal microbial flora is known through non-infection or disease-free microorganisms within or within the body. They protect and digest the skin, protect it against dangerous organisms that can cause infection or disease. Pathogens are called infection-causing microorganisms. Sometimes the factors that help spread the condition are called the cycle of infection. It is necessary to provide the infectious organ, infectious tank, exit portal, host, front door and move from tank to infectious person [9, 10].

2. Occupational health safety of radiography workers in the hospital

2.1 Infection exposure in in the hospital

It's not the infectious organism that transfers it from storage to recipients that interferes most directly with the infection cycle. To do so, the six main transmission routes should be understood. Direct contact is the first itinerary. This means that an infected person must contact the host and directly contact organisms with the sensitive tissue. For example, if an infectious organism contains the mucous membrane of an individual, syphilis, HIV infections may occur directly in the mucous membrane of a susceptible host [11, 12]. Furthermore, the frequent contact with staphylococcal and streptococcal patients is often associated with skin infections of hospital workers. The five other major paths of transmission are indirect and include transport of fluids, vectors, vehicles, airborne media, and droplets. An object of a pathogenic organism is known as a fomite. The catheter contaminated with urine is a typical example. Also included may be the x-ray table, Bucky vertical, image receptors, sponsor positioning with infectious fluids or, perhaps, gloves. Vectors are an arthropod whose organism develops or multiplies an infectious organism before it becomes a new host. Such infected patients can spread diseases to individuals. Examples of vectors include malaria- or dengue-carrying mosquitoes, bubonic fleas, and spotted fever spreading Lyrne or Rocky Mountain disease [13, 14]. Every vehicle with microorganisms is a medium. For example, contaminated food, water, medicines, or blood. The airborne air is contaminated either by five microns of dust or droplet nuclei (a micrometer, μm 0.001 mm) evaporated by an air-microorganism with long suspended air or by a smaller spore. Air currents and a sensitive host inhale these particles. Special air handling and ventilation is needed to avoid airborne transmission of these infected particles. M. Airborne infections include tuberculosis, rubeola, and varicella. Varicella may also contract these viruses by contacting vesicles. Goutlet contamination is usually experienced by host cough, sneezing, talking, or singing [15, 16]. Droplet transmission involves contact with susceptible person's large eye droplets, nose, and oral microorganisms with mucosal membranes. Unusually long, not air-suspended, 3 feet or less. Examples include influenza, meningitis, diphtheria, pertussis, pulmonary gout spread. Although many organisms may need constant warmth, humidity and concentration of nutrients, bacterial heating, cold and dry endosphorus. Endospores can float in poisonous corners awaiting an invading host. Bacterial spore-forming organisms cause serious but rare diseases like tetanus, anthrax, and botulism. Spores inhaled, eaten or contacted [17, 18]. The host provides moisture, warmth, and nutrients in an endocrine cell. Epidemiological studies show that for weeks, some viruses can resist drying at once. One case is that spores or viral infections cannot overestimate herpes virus cleanliness (orally and genitally).

Radiation exposure measures ionizing air by ionizing photon radiation, i.e. gamma and x-rays. it is defined as the power emitted by radiation within the given volume of air, divided by air mass [19].

2.2 The body's defense against infection

The three ways the human body is protected from invasion by microorganisms is to apply natural resilience and defense, resistance (also known as active immunity), and a temporary passive immune system. Mechanical barriers such as intact skin and mucous membranes are natural. Natural power. Natural power. Injuries such as severe burns, abrasion, and cuts can interfere with this skin protective barrier and increase infection risk. Respiratory, urinary, gastrointestinal and reproductive membranes trap foreign particles. The respiratory tract is also bordered by cilia carrying body mucus. Urinary tract is protected against increased urinary composition and external flow infections. Chemicals like lysozyme are also used to destroy invasive microorganisms in human tear, stomach, vagina, and skin acids [20].

Skin pH, salt, and dryness decrease the number of skin bacteria and prevent unwanted flora overgrowth. Nonetheless, microorganisms have access to the body. This results from daily activities like shaving and brushing [21].

This invasion begins with our second line, the inflammatory reaction. The flux of fluids and white blood cells through tissues increases blood flow to the site and allows swallowing and destroying invasive pathogens. That's called phagocytosis. When viruses infect the body, virus-infected cells create interferons, small protein molecules that protect non-infected cells and others from intrusion. Interferons are species-specific, currently in herpes and chronic hepatitis B and C treatment laboratories.

2.2.1 Acquired immunity

People are born with some immunity, but most people become disease resistant by becoming infected with a particular organism. This infection may or may not be an obvious disease. Immunity may also be granted from dead or weakened micro-organic strains infections or from inactivated toxin. This is known as immunity to some infection. Immunity is acquired because the body differs from the body 's foreign proteins. These substances are called antigens. Specific antigen-formed protein substances are antibodies. Antibodies. Antibodies B-cells, a white blood cell, are created to kill invasive alien substances with other white blood cells and avoid re-infection with that antigen. Because the body forms its own antibodies, it has long-term immunity.

2.2.2 Passive immunity

Passive immunity follows a specific infection with preformed antibodies. In this case, individuals receive pooled immune globulin (human blood and general population antibodies) before and after exposure to hepatitis A. Antibodies act promptly, but weaken over time to prevent disease. Neonate is temporarily immune to infections due to mother-to-fetus antibodies passing through the uterus. After birth, the infant continues to receive passive immunity. Since the body does not produce these antibodies, passive immunity is short-term [22].

2.3 Infectious diseases affected of the healthcare

Ergonomics investigates the working environment of the human body. In recent years, ergonomic awareness and training have reduced workplace injustice, but concern remains. The U.S. Labor Statistics Bureau reports hospital workers suffering similar injuries from industrial workers. The most commonly reported injuries are musculoskeletal disorders (MSDs). OSHA classified MSDs are sub-categories of recurrence motion injury (RMIs), repeated strain wound (RSIs), and cumulative trauma (CTDs). RMIs and RSIs, as their names suggest, result from repetitive or extensive pressure application. Stress from repetitive movement, excessive expansion, or long-term maintenance of the same position leads to muscle tissue-developing microtrauma. This microtrauma is the basis of cumulative trauma disorder, leading to chronic malaise and increased musculoskeletal lesions. CTD symptoms are pain, numbness, tingling, shyness, swelling, weakening, loss of function or overdeveloped muscle group (especially in hand and wrist). All health workers are at risk from lifting and moving patients and devices due to back strain. In addition, top neck and shoulders and rotating rashes often tighten the x-ray tube. Computerized technologists are more likely to experience spinal stress and RSI from intensive keyboard work. Intense keyboard work. RSI keyboard affects CTD 's hands and grips. Like tendinitis, carpal and ganglion syndrome. Imaging technologies, whose work takes longer to view the cathode ray tube monitor, also have vision problems. While ergonomic awareness is important for all employees, it's especially important for sonographers. RMIs and RSIs often affect Radiographer shoulder, arm, or wrist 80% of sonographers suffer work injuries. Sonographers number 80 percent. The root causes of these problems include equipment design, low posture, constant transducer pressure, difficult movements, unsatisfactory breaks, and overall stress. In recent years, high-end sonographic injuries have increased due to changes in equipment design and work characteristics [23].

Older transducers were heavier, but the patient had a stable arm that supported the transducer 's weight. New transductors are smaller and lighter, but their pressure and motor skills are needed. Furthermore, digital systems eliminated the need to change cassettes and process films to reduce activity. Imaging takes longer and specialization increases resemblance and recurrence. There are more tests; with techniques evolving, many tests are longer, harder and more repetitive. OSHA works with hospitals and equipment manufacturers to improve sonographic ergonomics, and education programs emphasize sonographers' role in postures, change positions, and breaks. Work injuries are minimized when enough equipment is available and properly used, and workers support each other. Frequent breaks and changes in position help minimize stress and position. Studies show that the right approach is continuing training programs and employer responses to employee ergonomic interests [6, 24].

2.4 Nosocomial infections

About 2 million patients are infected with nosocomial every year. Although many of these infections pose life-threats, CDC estimates that 90,000 people die from hospital-acquired infections every year and most of them are preventable. Medical conditions are ideal for developing and transmitting nosocomial infections. Typical sources of nosocomial infection include contaminated hands, instruments, and urinary catheters that facilitate microbes entering the body. Invasive methods allow pathogens to enter bloodstream and overcome patients' defensive mechanisms. The extensive and inappropriate use of wide-spectrum antibiotics has resulted in either hospital or community drug-resistant infections. Some of these infections can not be treated because they resist existing medicines. Developing a new medicinal product takes time, is expensive, and does not seem a lasting solution to this complex issue. Several nosocomial infections involve medical and multidrug-resistant patients. This means more than one antibiotic resistant. *Staphylococcus aureus* (MRSA) methicillin and enterococci resistant to vancomycin cause injury surgery, urinary tract and blood fluid infections. MRSA may also cause respiratory infections. Penicillin-resistant aeruginosa causes streptococcal and pseudomonas respiratory infection. The development and spread of these multi-drug-resistant infections was associated with antimicrobial overuse and poor infection management practices. Intensive infection control is required to reduce spread. These pathogens are hard to treat. Over the last 20 years, MRSA was recognized as a health problem. MRSA has been a community issue in recent years and is known as a community-related issue, or CA-MRSA. The CDC has created a relationship between new antibiotic use and sharing of personal contaminated objects, people in crowded environments, and poor hygiene. MRSA is associated with skin and soft tissue infections that can be treated with alternative antibiotics. These groups affected drug users, men who have sex with men, prisoners, military personnel, children in nursing facilities and athletes. Even when we write, other organisms adapt [2, 3, 17].

2.5 Management of occupational exposures to blood borne pathogens

If there is a sudden needle stick or a contaminated object breaks the skin, let the wound bleed under cold soap water. When the patient's body fluids sprinkle x-ray eyes, nose, or mouth, rinse your mucosal membranes with water. Even if the injury might seem trifling. In addition to the incident report, most hospitals now look for a baseline blood sample to prevent occupational infections. In addition, the health care provider will need to advise the X-ray technician on post-exposure prophylaxis (PEP) therapy after contaminated needle puncture. If treatment is recommended, it should take 2 hours for blood to become exposed. A four-week dos-drug regime is currently recommended for most PEP-defined HIV and several drug options. Hepatitis B and C are also tested using the x-ray HIV test. If radiologists have not used a vaccine for hepatitis B, the immune globulin and hepatitis B vaccines initiate immunity immediately. There is currently no effective hepatitis C therapy, therefore a follow-up HCV test is required to determine if the radiograph is exposed to a positive source. Because the blood cannot see HIV infection for about three months, it takes six months to get another HIV test [11, 17, 20].

2.6 Handling and disposal of contaminated

2.6.1 Handling linens

Objects or linens soiled with body secretions or excretions can be considered contaminated, but not visible, and can be used as fomites. The linen of every patient should be treated as lowly as possible. Place the edges of the linen in the center without throwing or flapping, and place balled linen immediately in the barrier to prevent contamination from the air. Most institutions today treat linen equally irrespective of the contamination. Place the linen in plastic bags, and use washing agents to prevent infection. Many hospitals offer hot water bags for cleaning, and laundry personnel process the linen several times [7, 9].

A modern hospital uses numerous devices to deliver contaminated waste, from simple objects such as cups and fabrics to complex objects such as catheterization. Contaminated disposal of waste only disposable items is used once, and then discarded. The only exception is that the same patient reuses the same non-sterile product immediately (e.g., the emesis basin). Each hospital has protocol for the disposal of devices. Some are split into containers covered with glass, plastic or paper, and others are combined. Follow procedure with x-rays. For disposal of objects contaminated with blood or liquid body, the Regulations require a biohazard symbol in the relevant container and marking. The needles and syringes used are placed in special, non-syringe recovery containers. New requirements for safer OSHA medical devices could reduce the high number of needle sticks that more unprotected, sharp workers had previously produced. There are lots of safe medical equipment. Some have a sheath to protect the contaminated needle, others have a needle which is retracting. When the needle is removed from the vein, the medical practitioner may take the needle back into the syringe. Use those safety features to avoid accidental needle sticks. When initial venous access is established, the needle-free system offers maximum needle stick protection and should be used in drugs and contrast media. Contaminated bandages and dressings are treated with gloves, they are directly sealed and disposed of in red plastic biohazard bags. Before being sent to the laboratory, place the specimens in safe containers and in a plastic bag marked with a biohazard symbol [21, 22].

2.6.2 Isolation technique

Before UP, diagnosis or suspected transmissible disease was the reason patients were isolated. All patients indicated that UP and BSP were potentially infectious. These new precautions were used in hospitals, in conjunction with their isolation policies. Hence, this text identifies several types of isolation systems previously used and describes the CDC recommendations as they stand. Initially, the hospital guidelines recommended one of two hospital systems: a category-specific system with seven different types of isolation, or a system specific to the disease. These two systems replace the current Guidelines. In addition to a synopsis of precautionary types and patients requiring precautions, Annex G is a CDC document reproducing reconciliations in order to prevent hospital isolations [3, 9, 12].

2.6.3 Transmission-based precautions

The CDC has recommended that patients be isolated by transmission precautions as part of the standard precautions. This system replaces precautions for older categorized diseases that are based on transmission. These sets aim to minimize airborne transmission, droplets and risk of contact. They can be used individually or with standard precautions, on a number of disease pathways [4, 9].

2.6.4 Airborne precautions

Airborne precautions aim to reduce the risk of transferring infectious or gout nuclei particles (5 ppm or less) to a susceptible person. They take airborne precautions to prevent tuberculosis and rubeola. Medical professionals and visitors in a room of an infectious person must wear NIOSH-approved particulate breathers. These masks must filter 1 micron with an efficiency of 95 percent. Patients undergo airborne treatment in rooms with negative airflows and special air circulation, with more than six external air interchanges per hour or via HEPA filters. These rooms are forever closed [3, 7].

2.6.5 Droplet precautions

Droplet precautions have been designed to reduce sensitive nose or mouth contact with particles of large droplet connectivity (over 5 microns). Precautions are applied to prevent transmission of diseases such as diphtheria, pneumonia, and influenza. Medical staff and visitors in contact with these patients must wear surgical masks but they do not require special circulation of air in these rooms. Contact precautions are designed to minimize the risk of pathogen transmission through direct skin-to-skin contact, or indirect contact with a contaminated object. Contact precautions are used to prevent MRSA- and new VRE-resistant infections. (H7:0157) Coli. It must be worn by doctors in close contact with infected patients who cause gastrointestinal and renal problems and various sunlike infections such as glove, and clothing. Contact precautions when merging airborne. Airborne and contact precautions are combined to minimize the risk of airborne droplet nodes transmitting pathogens and direct contact with the skin. These precautions are used to prevent the spread of the chicken pox and herpes zoster by SARS and varicella viruses. Health care workers without a pox should avoid contact with patients who are infected. Infected personnel do not need to have any masks beforehand [7, 9, 23].

2.7 Radiography of isolation patients

Using friendly patient interest in protective radiation functions and avoiding fear or repulsion, radiographers can help alleviate those sensations. Isolation Two patients require x-rays, two rays preferred. Patient belongs to the 'dirty' team, and the device is managed by the 'clean' Member. Although both radiographers must take all the prescribed isolation precautions, the 'clean' member does not have direct contact with the patient, bed or any item that the patient may have touched. Only the X-ray machine and uncovered image receptors (IR) use this radiogram. This team method minimizes contamination with the x-rays, which is difficult to disinfect completely. Radiographer and his colleagues shall prepare the required IRs before entering the insulation room by putting each in a smoothly fitting plastic bag and the lead table of Don Radiographer. The jewelry should be removed from the x-ray, view it in the pocket or pin it in the uniform of the x-ray [9, 12, 25].

At the door, radiographer shall take the necessary precautions (e.g., gloves, dresses, and masks). Apply the recommended guidelines for isolation and donate protective clothing for the specified type of isolation. It can be carried out in a hallway adjacent to the area in which the room is isolated. Now the radiographers are ready to go to bed. Welcome to the procedure, explain, and introduce yourself. The dirty team member places the IR properly, so that the exposure side is toward the radiation tube. Team cleaner locates the machine and displays controls. After each exposure has finished, the IR is recovered with partial deletion of the protective cover. It then offers an edge-clean teammate. The contaminated cover is placed in the appropriate container which keeps the IR in the cabinet of the engine. The radiology technologist must make sure the patient is safe and comfortable, before removing the x-ray dress at the end of the test. Radiology technologist must firstly remove the gloves [13, 15, 26].

2.8 Precautions for compromised patients

The immunity of the patient is very limited, and it takes special precautions to prevent inflammation. Organ transplants may be received, along with immunosuppressive medicines. The burning of patients and neonates may also require these precautions. Patients undergoing chemotherapy sometimes use these precautions to reduce resistance. Once this is called reverse isolation, or isolation from protection. The 1983 Federal Isolation Directive removed the protection class, mainly because it differs in purpose and procedure from other categories I of isolation. The basics are identical! Those terms may still be used in the clinical environment by the radiograph. Precautions for an affected patient require that the equipment be cleaned before they enter the room. Hand hygiene is required before the patient touches the bed or the patient's items. Masks, caps, sterile robes and handkerchiefs can be worn as an operation or modified. Modified technique leads to very high sterile-protocol aseptic medical therapy. Specific precautions are taken outside of the room for patients. Team member is the "clean" X-ray that puts the patient under guard. This X-ray user avoids contact with uncovered IRs, X-rays and other potentially contaminated objects using the right protective clothing. This X-ray folds the edges, keeping it open if the second X-ray is to properly cover the IR inside the sterile cassettlement. It's important that there is no contamination outside the cover. The patient, bed, clean object and IR only affect the clean x-ray and only the filtered x-ray affects the device. That is precisely the opposite of isolation.

3. Conclusion

In this chapter, we defined aseptic medical systems as a means of reducing and interfering with the process of spreading pathogenic microorganisms across the environment. Operational asepsis however constitutes destruction of equipment or spores and organisms for patient care. In the first case, sterile linen, gloves, and surgical devices are examples, but many other operations require sterile treatment, such as lumbar perforations, catheterization, and injections, as well as some patients who are immunocompromised. Too few naked microorganisms are visible, like bacteria, protozoa, prions, and fungi [2, 3]. Some microorganisms protect and benefit individuals and are called normal flora: some are hazardous, cause disease and infection, and are known to be pathogenic. The infectious organism, infection tank, exit and entry portals, transmission mode and sensitive home are all part of the infectious cycle. Include body protection in three ways: resistance, defense, immunity, short-term immunity, and microorganism infestations. Body protection includes factors propagating disease. New diseases, existing effects or geographical conditions, and repeated old diseases caused by old diseases or mutated diseases are the emerging conditions. Emerging diseases are a major issue. Many factors can lead to emerging diseases, including increased exposure to vectors, population growth, migration to crowded cities, global travel, antimicrobial overuse, public safety crashes, and biological terror [7, 8]. The total number of cases in the U.S. and worldwide continues to increase. HIV/AIDS is a major public health issue. MSM and IDUs are the most common cases. Transmission routes include sex, infected blood, body and needle fluids, placenta, fetal mother, and breast-milk babies. As a blood borne pathogen, transmission risk to health workers is very low. The main concerns are health workers, both bloodborne and diagnosed with hepatitis B and C. 0 Vaccines and preventive therapies, but C is not available. Medical workers are less likely to contract C, but you get more chronic liver infection and cirrhosis. Contamination of feces and water transmits A and E. Hepatitis A is the disease's most common vaccine. If needles are infected with the patient's eye needle, nose, or mouth splashes with the patient's fluid, post-exposure healthcare practitioners should use procedures. Tuberculosis is primarily M-induced pulmonary disease. Air pollution and tuberculosis. Foreign-born residents are America is most common. Tuberculin skin testing is the easiest way to test TB infection. Real TB hospitals must undergo procedures such as tuberculin skin testing, personal breathing facilities, one or more negative air pressure and special ventilation isolation rooms. Aseptic therapy aims to reduce transmission risk to sensitive people of infectious organisms. Frequent hand hygiene is the best aseptic practice [1, 2, 23]. Hand hygiene includes soap and water washing your hands, taking spumes or gels if no visible soil is present. Good household management reduces airborne infections and pathogens. Examples of possible forms of medical aseptic include dust, disinfection, and good liner management, dry and wet waste disposal, and sharp container use. Current isolation and infection management policies have evolved in home quarantining families. Initially, infection was only diagnosed in isolated patients, but HIV and AIDS changed. Besides infectious diseases, new treatment processes were introduced for all patients in hospitals. The current system has two areas: (1) Defense and hygiene barriers are standard precautions for all patients based on patient contact. (2) Transmission-based precautions apply to patients with infectious diseases [13, 26].

Health workers must wear protective clothing, regardless of patient contact. Airborne, droplet and contact transmission risk can be reduced independently or in combination by using three categories of precautions. The isolating patient's x-rays involve two individuals: (1) the x-rays are placed as "clean x-rays" (2) the receptive image is "dirty" and the patient as infectious. If they remember their roles, cross-contamination is minimized. Both X-rays give the inspection and testing room clothing. X-rays are carefully removed, imaging, recording equipment disinfected, and hand hygiene after testing is done. Radiology Department may refer isolated patients for imaging studies [23, 24]. To wear protective clothing and work as a team to complete the exam, at least two radiation are needed. The first is patient placement, and the second is equipment placement and control. After transportation, the stretcher or wheelchair is covered in paper. The linen, wet and dry waste should be properly disinfected in the X-ray room. Immunosuppression requires safeguards for endangered patients, including weakened immune systems, drugs, brandy, and neonates [17, 19]. The patient is in control as "clean ray" and "dirty." Easy hands smooth clothing, gloves and sterile clothing are safeguards. All organisms, spores, and procedures, including aseptic surgical disease, must be destroyed. Operational aseptics are often surgery-related but also used when an invasive procedure such as lobster punctures or urinary catheterization is performed. Aseptic surgical therapy also treats patients with immune problems. Operations involve sterile fields, operational sprinkling, and invasive clothing. Four different sterilization techniques and equipment can be used for chemical, dry, ethylene-oxide gas, plasma gas and autoclave. Each method recommends advantages, disadvantages, and uses. Sterility and biological indicators are reused to ensure that all packages are properly sterilized, damaging all forms of microbial life during sterilization. Micro-organisms can use sterile fields without sterile equipment. Sterility and supply of the packet must be adequately confirmed and opened before establishing a sterile field to prevent contamination. If a sterile field is established, additional sterile objects and liquids may follow suitable procedures [12, 24].

Acknowledgements

I would like to express my gratitude toward Dr. Yousif Abdallah (y.yousif@mu.edu.sa) associate professor of radiology, Majmaah university for providing the necessary support and assistance for completing this chapter.

Author details

Hasna Albander
Medical Physicist Department, Prince Sultan Military Medical City Riyadh, Riyadh, Saudi Arabia

*Address all correspondence to: hasna_bb@hotmail.com

References

[1] Amersham Health X-Ray Products: Clinical references, glucophage (metformin) and iodinated contrast media, pp 5-7.

[2] Abdallah Y. An Introduction to PACS in Radiology Service: Theory and Practice. Vol. 2. Berlin, Germany: LAP LAMBERT Academic Publishing; 2012. pp. 140-153

[3] ASRT Task Force on Governance Restructuring: Recommended governance structure, November 2002, pp 1-6.

[4] Abdallah Y, Yousef R. Augmentation of X-rays images using pixel intensity values adjustments. International Journal of Science and Research (IJSR). 2015;4 (2):pp.2425-2430

[5] Bonewit-West K: Clinical procedures for medical assistants, ed 7, Philadelphia, 2008, WB Saunders Bracco imaging pharmaceutical products, contrast media Centers for Disease Control and Prevention: Division of Health Care Quality Promotion: Surveillance of health care personnel with HIV/AIDS as of 2001.

[6] Abdallah Y. Application of Analysis Approach in Noise Estimation, Using Image Processing Program. Germany: Lambert Publishing Press GmbH & Co. KG; 2011. pp. 123-125 [4]

[7] Centers for Disease Control and Prevention: Division of Tuberculosis Elimination: Core curriculum on tuberculosis, ed 4, 2000, Chapter 4-Testing for TB disease and infection.

[8] Abdallah Y. History of medical imaging. Archives of Medicine and Health Sciences. 2017;5:275-278

[9] Centers for Disease Control and Prevention: Exposure to blood: what health-care workers need to know, 2002, pp 1-8.

[10] Centers for Disease Control and Prevention: Guidelines for hand hygiene in health-care settings, MMWR Morb Mortal Wkly Rep 51IRR-2002:16:l-44,.

[11] Centers for Disease Control and Prevention: Guideline for Isolation Precautions: Preventing Transmission of Infectious Agents in Healthcare Settings 2007, Part 11, Fundamental elements needed to prevent transmission of infectious agents in healthcare settings, June 2007.

[12] Centers for Disease Control and Prevention: HIV/AIDS surveillance report, 2005, vol. 17, Reved, Atlanta: U.S. Department of Health and Human Services, CDC, 1-54, 2007.

[13] Centers for Disease Control and Prevention: Reported tuberculosis in the United States, 2006, Atlanta: U.S. Department of Health and Human Services, CDC, October 2007.

[14] Abdallah Y. An Introduction to PACS in Radiology Service: Theory and Practice. LAP LAMBERT Academic Publishing. Berlin, Germany. 2012:2. 140-153

[15] Abdallah Y. and Abuhadi N. The Role of Magnetic Resonance Imaging (MRI) in Autonomic Nervous System Monitoring, Autonomic Nervous System Monitoring - Heart Rate Variability, IntechOpen:2019. pp.125-137

[16] Centers for Disease Control and Prevention: Synopsis of types ofprecautions and patients requiring theprecautions, February 1997.

[17] Centers for Disease Control and Prevention: Trends in tuberculosis morbidity-United States, 1992-2002, MMWR Morb Mortal Wkly Rep. 2003:52(11):217-222,

[18] Chobanian AV et al: The Seventh Report of the Joint National Committee on Prevention, Detection, Evaluation, and Treatment of High Blood Pressure, JAMA, 289(19):2560-2572,2003.

[19] Abdallah Y. and Abuhadi N. Entrance Skin Dose Measurement for Diagnostic Spinal Radiographic Examinations in King Khalid Hospital, Saudi Arabia: A Prospective Study, Journal of clinical and Diagnostic Research, 2020;3(14):pp.

[20] Durand KS: Critical thinking: developing skills in radiography, Philadelphia, 1999, FA Davis.
Elkin MK, Perry AG, Potter PA: Nursing interventions and clinical skills, ed 4, St Louis, 2007, Mosby.

[21] Enrollment snapshot of radiography, radiation therapy and nuclear medicine programs, 2019, ASRT.

[22] Abdallah Y. Introduction to dental Radiography: Theory and Practice. Vol. 2. Berlin, Germany: LAP LAMBERT Academic Publishing; 2018. pp. 120-133

[23] Abdallah Y. A short Textbook on Care of patient in Radiotherapy Department. Berlin, Germany: LAP LAMBERT Academic Publishing; 2018. pp. 120-133

[24] Frank E, Long B, Smith B: Merrill's atlas of radiographic positions and radiologic procedures, ed 11, St Louis,2007, Mosby.

[25] Furlow B: Ergonomics in the health care environment, Journal of the American Society of Radiologic Technologists 2002.74(2):137-150.

[26] Abdallah Y, Abdullah, E, Alqahtani T, Abuhadi N, Study of a five years survival rate of cancer in Sudanese, Oncology and Radiotherapy, 14: (3): 2020: 022-025.

Chapter 6

Characterization of Brain Stroke Using Image and Signal Processing Techniques

Abdullah Alamoudi and Yousif Abdallah

Abstract

Cross-sectional imaging approaches play a key role in assessing bleeding brain injuries. Doctors commonly determine bleeding size and severity in CT and MRI. Separating and identifying artifacts is extremely important in processing medical images. Image and signal processing are used to classify tissues within images closely linked to edges. In CT images, a subjective process takes a stroke 's manual contour with less precision. This chapter presents the application of both image and signal processing techniques in the characterization of Brain Stroke field. This chapter also summarizes how to characterize the brain stroke using different image processing algorithms such as ROI based segmentation and watershed methods.

Keywords: brain stroke, image processing, signal processing

1. Introduction

A medical condition called a stroke is cell death associated with weak blood flow into the brain. It is an ischemic stroke caused by insanity caused by blood flow, and it is a bleeding that in two different forms causes hemorrhagic stroke. Both have helped to prevent the proper functioning of brain sections [1–7]. The World Health Organization has indicated that it is known as a neurological impairment by cerebral vascular factor as a stroke in the 1970s. One of the most common types of stroke is ischemia which causes a loss of brain functions because of severe lack of blood supply [8–11]. Because there are treatments that can reduce the severity of stroke symptoms if given early enough, many people now prefer the more urgent wording "stroke" or "acute ischemic stroke (AIS)" over the less urgent "brain attack" and "acute ischemic stroke" [12–19]. The headaches caused by this disease can be severe and they may cause strokes. In a stroke, symptoms might include possible partially done strokes. Problems that can arise, if an e-cigarette is not used properly, include bladder sickness and bladder dysfunction. High blood pressure of the veins is the most important risk factor on stroke. The risk of the disease falls on other risk factors, such as smoking, obesity, elevated blood cholesterol, diabetes, and hypertension [20–24]. Diagnosis is usually based on the clinical investigation and is assisted by medical imaging, such as CT or MRI scans [25–29]. CT scans may rule out bleeding, but ischemia, which usually does not appear early in the CT scan, may not necessarily be excluded [30–33]. Other tests are performed to identify risk factors and to rule out other possible causes, such as electrocardiogram (ECG) and blood tests [34–37]. Aspirin may be used to prevent clots from forming on the inside of the blood vessel walls. Statins may be used to prevent clots from forming within your blood vessels. For small areas of injury, clot removal may be performed. Stroke reminiscence may also be performed to create a place where the brain can begin again with stroke recovery. If your brain is injured, a surgically placed clot of another substance may be used to stop bleeding in the parts of the brain that are injured [7, 38]. Personal computer with suitable software can use to modify and custom a digital image algorithm. A personal computer can produce your own customized digital image. Digital image processing, as opposed to analog signal processing, has many advantages. The new software has characteristics that allow one to be more flexible with visually, audio and text output features. Because digital image processing can be modeled in a multidimensional way, digital images can be defined as two (or more) dimensional. In 1972, EMI Hounsfield, (a gentleman engineer) calculated subtle methods to immerse a radiolucent X-ray tube into a potable medium which was used to take images within patients' heads (computer tomography). In order to construct a cross-section of the entirety of an image, the CT scanner is established on the basis of the anatomy of the human body. In 1975, EMI demonstrated a full body scanner with a cross-sectional scan in order to identify body parts and other people in the body. The Nobel Prize is earned by this type of research in 1979. In the 1990s, medical image processing technologies were used to control heart rates during coronary artery bypass grafts [17, 24].

2. Stroke classification

These two types of strokes, Ischemic and Hemorrhagic, have different properties. They are caused by a stroke, and the damage that stroke brings to brain. Besides, the infections that cause meningitis are caused when blood vessels burst or leaks out of the body. 87% of stroke pain is due to a reduced blood supply to the brain, and the rest is due to bleeding. Some people living in ischemic areas might feel some internal bleeding. This is a cause of poor blood flow in the walls of the heart [2, 39].

Strokes that are the result of ischemic damage to the brain can be caused. In order to answer this question, one will need to weigh four different points of view:

1. First, a blood clot could form (obstruction of a blood vessel by a blood clot forming locally)

2. Myocardial infarction [Which causes blockages to the blood vessels in the heart].

3. Local conditions with low levels of circulation affect other areas of the body, causing widespread blood pressure changes.

4. Brain veins are an area of venous thrombosis [22, 40].

Acute Ischemic Strokes (IS) has a myriad of classifications. The most common one is Cryptogenic stroke. it comprises the usual cause for this type of stroke which makes up about 30–40 percent of all ischemic strokes. The number of IS strokes is about 1,500,000 per year. Depending on the level of symptoms, the Oxford Community stroke program (SCAP) consists of symptomatic or refractory (traumatic) strokes; these experiences are considered to be kind of those seen in severe stroke; the Mini–Mental state exam, or the McIntosh Edinburgh assessment; the total anterior circulation, or lacuna infarction; or secondary circulatory event is an integral part of the Oxford Community stroke program, therefore, the focal branch infarction, or focal ischemic attack or stroke; and the changes in mental, depending on the amount of signs and symptoms of the Oxford Community stroke program (SCAP), and the Oxford Community stroke program (SCAP); those mentioned are the "Oxford Community stroke program", the "Oxford Community stroke program" attack! (POCI). The level of the stroke, the area of the brain affected, the symptoms and prognosis are defined by the following four groups; [24, 25] The TOAST classification (Orga Stroke Assay 10172 Acute Stroke Therapy) is dependent on clinical symptoms and the outcomes of further investigations [41–43]. Good thing is that a stroke is known to be partly caused by particular risk factors, such as thrombosis or embolism of arteriosclerosis or stroke [27, 44–47].

There are two types of strokes that cause bleeding: hemorrhagic and ischemic.

1. It specifically affects the brain, as it has life-threatening consequences (when an artery in the brain bursts, flooding the surrounding tissue with blood).

2. Bleeding is typically seen on the outside of the brain tissue and between the arachnoid and the pia mater. Falling may cause a subarachnoid hemorrhage (the delicate innermost layer of the three layers of the meninges that surround the brain).

There are different types of bleeding, one of which is ablated. There are also two primary kinds of intracranial hemorrhages, which are also called "bleeding" or "bleeding." Included under that are two forms of "bleeding" called "hematoma," which is a type of subdural hematoma. The "whole" of this document is worded confusingly. It says "'hematoma" is also included under" 'bleeding." It should read "Also, there are two different kinds of hemorrhagic strokes..." [48–51].

2.1 Stroke signs and symptoms

On the contrary, stroke symptoms often arrive without prior warning. When you see these symptoms, it's probably not going to be long before they become noticeable. In some cases, symptoms vary in different brain areas because of an infection. This disease has more effect in larger parts of the brain, meaning that the loss of neural features will likely be more costly. In addition, there are different signs that may lead to strokes. This part of the patient may compress in the location of the bleeding, such as in intracranial bleeding. For some people who have certain types of stroke, headaches are not always associated with their stroke. For example, subarachnoid hemorrhage and cerebral thrombosis are strokes that sometimes cause headaches [36, 52, 53].

If it uses the main central pathways that the brain is involved with, it will work. When we look at a specific test, we can find that its one of the three pathways we use can fail.

1. Parkinsonism and a very tenuous facial muscles are seen.

2. Target specificity of

3. Feelings of companionship, enhancement, and calmness.

4. Many of the symptoms of breast cancer include intense muscle spasms, increased reflectivity and a gradual weakening of muscles due to loss of control [54].

Most of the time, symptoms on one side of the body are involved (unilateral). Since the damage to the brain is always located in another hemisphere, it affects the non-damaged side of the brain instead of the damage side. Although some signs may be caused by bumps in the legs, such as leg pain, it is absolutely clear that any serious injury can affect all of these symptoms. Therefore, to approach whether or not there is also a symptom that is not definite is difficult. To man into. Therefore, the part of the brain that is damaged by the stroke can cause deficits in the following cranial nerve functions:

1. There are changes in the sense of smell, taste or sight in addition to the other senses (total or partial)

2. The "Paranoia" side effect can cause the eyes to twitch, or tremble, as well as causing wornness or weakness in the eye muscles.

3. Remove, try to resist from swallowing, reduce pupil size, like escape.

4. A reduction in facial cranes and movement, often leading to emotional swings.

5. Nystagmus and balance problems can occur.

6. Breathing or heart rate changes occur.

7. The weakness of the muscles is due to the incomplete development of the right side of the heart.

8. A decline in the oral health (inability to stick out the tongue or move it from side to side) [55–58].

2.1.1 Stroke symptoms

1. This is also called aphasia (difficulty with verbal expression, hearing comprehension, reading and writing; typically involved in the field of Broca or Wernicke)

2. An after effect of being mentally ill (motor speech disorder resulting from neurological injury)

3. Dyslexia is usually a problem (altered voluntary movements)

4. The visual field might be abnormal.

5. Memory impairments are common (involvement of temporal lobe)

6. He's a very angry man. A madman (involvement of parietal lobe)

7. A naked brain, nervy, insecure, and sexually hyperactive is intense of a person (with involvement of frontal lobe)

8. The brain's function may become compromised if it is dealt a moderate stroke.

If the cerebellum is busy and working well, a person will have ataxia.

1. A public walkway or public sidewalk.

2. Some of the plans have changed.

3. Lack of necessary resources [59–62].

2.2 Stroke causes

2.2.1 Thrombotic stroke

When a child has a thrombosis, there is typically a plaque deposit around the blockage. Stroke may not be as serious as a heart attack, since the blood pressure may not necessarily drop like in a heart attack. It is an embolism in the heart (see below). This medication, applied to a vein, could lead to the development of a blood clot, as this may make the blood flow less freely. Both types of stroke can result in a pronounced stroke.

- The internal carotid artery, like the rest of the arteries in the human body, has tighter associations with vascular disease, especially in the back and neck. Coronary artery disease, peripheral vascular disease (PVD) atherosclerosis, vasoconstriction, atherosclerotic disease of arteries of various kinds, and varying inflammatory diseases affecting the walls of vessels (Takayasu arteritis, g).

- The small vascular thrombosis disorders consist of a few different diseases that may damage the internal workings of the body. These diseases include small, placental inside the blood flow: lipohyalinosis (a buildup of fatty hyaline in blood vessels), and a mutation [63, 64].

2.2.2 Embolic stroke

The reason why a stroke occurs is because a clot gets in the blood vessels. The doctor will give you some medication (a blockage of an artery). There were many blood clots found in the different vessels, with these being composed of the most of them being blood fat cells and bacterial accumulations. It is always important to be able to locate and stop the clot. Patients who have this disease may start to experience symptoms within just a couple of weeks after the symptoms appear. These symptoms can be just as intermittent as the embolus re-routes elsewhere or goes back empty. The nail used in this study may also be applicable to patients with coronary artery disease (CAD) and atrial fibrillation (AF) [44].

With stroke, the heart, brain, and blood vessels each need to be evaluated separately [65].

1. High risk candidates include patients with atrial fibrillation or paroxysmal atrial fibrillation, sick sinus syndrome, chronic myocardial infarction (heart attack), mitral or aortic valve disease and those with known atrial or ventricular thrombus.

2. Systolic impulses are completely blocked by a left ventricular aneurysm in coronary atherosclerotic heart disease history; aneurysm atrial septal. Athletes may be treated if they have: PFO and left atrial aneurysm; atrial aneurysm and/or patent aneurysm; patent foramen ovum and atrial aneurysm; left ventricular aneurysm and/or heart muscle aneurysm; left atrial aneurysm or triple atrial complex aneurysm.

If a stroke occurs on the same side of the body, it predicts that the risk of a stroke will be 1% a year. The cause of stroke in this kind of patients is past a particular form of the disease (ESUS). The subtypes of cryptogenic stroke. The first part is likely that one of the ischemic strokes will be [65–67].

2.2.3 Cerebral hypoperfusion

When the brain is not given enough blood supply, it is called mild corto-cortical hypoperfusion. Sometimes, part of the brain is lost to various circumstances, such as a someone being concussed. Heart diseases, such as a recent heart attack, is a common health concern. This is the reason. For the purpose of. According to the studies, all areas of the brain has grown and is now much larger. However, at some point it might seem small, like compressed. Development and the brain It is a form of heart attack called water fall. When the brain is under a lot of strain, blood can cease from flowing at the pained area, and brain damage can be caused. When the brain is in a stress condition, brain activity will be reduced or stifled. The cerebral venous sinus is not only dangerous for forming clots in the brain, but also dangerous for how it raises blood pressure. This type of stroke is much more likely than any other type of stroke [22]. Strokes can occur to the brain or to the arteries because of a damage that can take place in either location. There are a number of potential causes to understand in this patient setup. The possibility of a medical condition present is the most likely to be possible cause (e.g., amphetamines or cocaine). The blood cells migrate to the ventricle in an unhealthy state. Preventing this can prevent tumor cells from becoming engorged. About a third of the ventricles are not being used by the brain. Within 30 days of an intracerebral hemorrhage, at least a 40% survival rate is possible and higher than that of other neurodegenerative diseases and subarachnoid hemorrhages (which technically may also be classified as a type of stroke [68, 69]). Heart attacks can also result from other conditions that occur, due to the heart attack itself. Most likely, cocaine is the reason behind an increase in crack use [49].

2.2.4 Silent stroke

Apart from damage, this disease also has several silent strokes that can cause long-term brain damage. Tests have shown that silent strokes can sometimes lead to a disease in the future. All people who have experienced a major stroke are also susceptible to having a silent, milder stroke. The lifetime risk of having a stroke is slightly higher than the odds of getting killed during a car accident. Of the 770,000 strokes, about half of them were symptomatic strokes such as blood clots, and 11 million were strokes, hemorrhages, or MRI infarctions. Injury detection by such a system, which is so advanced, often is not noticed. Those strokes that are diagnosed as silent occur five times more often than those strokes that are fatal. When the body is working out, it is automatically producing the malodorous by-product of metabolism, the infamous lactic acid. Acidosis occurs when too much acid is produced, which can interfere with the normal functioning of the mind. Since this is an area in which the industry demonstrated great innovation, with fat in the form of ethersys which continued to cause companies to pull billions of dollars of income from emerging markets their findings were thereafter patented. They made patents filings which include the discovery of a variety of new compounds related to adenosine which leads them to prevent competitors from successfully copying the source of revenue (ATP). The part of town is referred to as simply "Mid" because it is inconveniently located. Glutamate binds to receptors to tear down the neurons. Neural ion homeostasis is usually maintained by a few rare plants. This stroke reduces the value, making it harder to chip off the paint, damaging the microscopic paint. In that case, high levels of glutamate are sequestered in the cytoplasm.

The elevated levels of chemical glutamate cause calcium to enter cells. A series of chain reactions in mitochondria and lack of sufficient oxygen over time leads to a steady accumulation of free radicals and reactive oxygen species. When we have finished digesting and removing cellular and extracellular material. There are several potential problems with the interior of the ship. Antioxidants are only effective in the endothelium and do NOT work in the brain itself. Free radicals are involved in cell death, but so is life. The brain is particularly sensitive to lack of blood supply [70–74].

The plasma membrane of damaged cells can lose its blood supply and be unable to uptake oxygen and much needed nutrients. In addition, inflammation can cause damage the overlying brain. It is capable of other possible proteolytic actions. It is possible for severe brain or head injuries to occurs due to a loss of cerebral vascular integrity, or to a case of dangerous stroke. Diseases that cause hemorrhagic strokes have causes that are still being investigated. There are many possible causes of a stroke, such as high blood pressure, aneurysm, a vascular fistula, arterial disease of the carotid artery, and an allergic reaction. When using the e-cigarette, people can have minor damage in the brain due to a lack of blood flow to the brain [61, 74–78].

2.3 Stroke diagnosis

MRI and CT scans are used to determine the amount of brain damage caused when a stroke occurs. The imaging methods allowed the phenomenon of occultation to be located. Scanning techniques can help identify a stroke's subtype and identify where its source is. Doctors may also be able to perform other blood tests that can help diagnose a stroke as well. Blood tests can reveal what something is really like to another person [62].

2.3.1 Physical examination

A medical examination involves cross-referencing a person's past medical history to their current clinical history. If there is a normal level of stroke severity, it is recommended to assign a normal level.

2.3.2 Imaging

The case study: "Ischemic stroke" [63].

- An x-ray of the chest (without contrast enhancements)
    - Recovery Time: (less than 10 percent within first 3 hours of symptom onset)
    - Specificity of positive predictive value = 96%.
- On the MRI scans.
    - Affectivity is, well, very strong.
    - Specificity of objects (98%).
- When it comes to diagnosing head injury in the hospital, it's important to use.
    - It's a type of MRI scan for NMA (without contrast enhancements)
    - The sensitivity dropped by eleven percent.

- o Ultrasound scans are used.
- o the level of sensitivity is 83 percent.
- o Personalization is complete.

The MRI scan is sufficient to be evaluated for a chronic stroke. However, it may also be necessary for scanning with SPECT or PET. The metabolism of PET, brain blood movement isotopes, PET, and PET neurons are reported as PET and SPECT. In the blood supply, CT scans identify mild ischemic strokes with tender detection of blight. To estimate the underlying cause of a CT test, it is possible to use many other image enhancers. Determination of the quality of these medicines is very important, depending on the prescription. The selection of the stroke response will depend heavily on the cause of the stroke. The conventional way is the following:

- Doppler Ultrasound Studies (for detection or pre-brain diagnosis of carotid stenosis);
- The electrocardiogram or echocardiogram (ECG) (for identification of arrhythmias and after cardiac clots may spread to brain vessels throughout the bloodstream)
- Survey for the detection of abnormal rhythms of the heart.
- Cerebral vasculature angiography, in which bleeding is presumed to be due to aneurysm or arteriovenous malformation.
- Blood tests to evaluate the presence of high blood cholesterol or whether it could be a rare process, including, etc. There are abnormal tests for blood.

If hemorrhagic stroke test deficiencies are present, the CT or MRI contrast scan can identify cerebral artery deformation or any other source of bleeding or structural MRI if this does not result (for example, aneurysms). Invasive cerebral angiography may also be performed if the underlying cause of bleeding is not identified but implies access to the blood stream with the intravascular catheter, which can cause additional strokes and complications at the place of insertion, and therefore this study is reserved for certain situations [65].

2.3.3 Misdiagnosis

The diagnosis ranges from 2 to 27 per cent of ischemic stroke cases. A stroke that has other characters is the 'Chameleon stroke.' Failure to diagnose people without a stroke also has the potential. One to two percent of the total is typically one to two percent of the penile bleeder that produces intracerebral bleeding through thrombosis addiction (one to two percent, less in stroke). The cost of medical treatment is helped by this superfluous treatment. However, the AHA/ASA advice suggests that further studies should delay intravenous tPA treatment [67]. African Americans, Latin Americans, Asians, and Pacific Islanders are more likely to be misrepresented for a condition other than stroke when they have a stroke. Moreover, women younger than 44 are 7 times more likely than people older than 75 years of age to have a stroke. For younger trauma sufferers, this can be the case [66]. Experimental studies in other medical centers have shown that hyperacute RMI m is hyperacute [66].

3. Medical imaging processing for stroke

Doctors have multiple strategies and methods for identifying medical images to diagnose diseases. Cell segmentation in diseases, with the help of MATLAB, can be the easiest way for doctors to examine illnesses of the immoral tissue. Image classification in sectors with structural units is the interpretation and analysis of an image that you plan to be mutually compatible. The MI brain imaging is one of the most competitive physiques in the organism, so explaining brain segmentation is a detailed assignment of which the assistant will not work because... Biomedical imagery represents the body that consists of the soft tissue, organ, and bone structure. In such circumstances, they cannot tell whether or not this raw biomedical view of adolescent health climaxes. This means that biomedical image analysis through image handling is so critical that it is essential for medics to be conscious of special problems and of their development related to disease and growth problems. There are numerous types of medical visual sectors in MATLAB application like threshold and morphology [5, 12]. Morphological and philological methods are forms of different pictures for some brain strokes. The simplest and the most frequently identified technique in the pixel is to decide that for all pixels measured below a given point above or below intensity it would form part of a pixel. Form processing requires a morphological work. This combines two different morphological procedures, expansion, and exhaustion. With a dilate, center activation, or for the active expansion of pixel, with erosion of their neighbors is the minimum and, at a minimum, the minimum required to accommodate its neighbors. The two activities are linear as well. They are not settings of rotatable transitions which usually result in an unusual image from each of them, one after another. It's used to prevent background defects from deepension to dilation (Opening). However, by closing small gaps [5, 6], to compensate the shape of the object, erosion dilation will also be used to fill small gaps. It becomes the U.S.'s fourth major cause of death in the United States that kills people every four min. More then00,000 people who experienced a stroke arise from respiratory complications in the brain (a bloodstream blocks) or from the spotted blood vessel. The level of brain improvement, for example, increased owing to an increase in medical malpractice. This has in many ways culminated in an appropriate medical diagnosis. However, it is not simple to correctly detect an incident. In this document we seek to articulate a conceptual process to help physicians deal with illnesses on a social basis. Skin rash was detected through image purchase selectivity. In order to evaluate brain stroke images from magnetic resonance imaging, the examiner uses the MATLAB panel (MRI).

Many scientists such as [11, 12, 35, 56, 71–74] described in this paper, Diagnostic Application of Brain Image Processing and the System of Stroke Analysis, that, particularly relative to standard MRI technologies are generally used for early examination and therapy of vaccines. This study aims at using the photographic editing that can effectively measure volume strength and provide 3D evidence of damage restructuring with a sound analysis system, assisted by software technicians. Add on that. Our system envisages increased accuracy in the design and interpretation of acute stroke damage, longer calculation time and volume, and a 3D repair plan that will make doctors simpler for dealing with and better evaluating patients, as well as to treat them better. The study findings have shown that this suggested system is better efficient than the existing technique, so this system is therefore also an efficiency. The case study also illustrated through a quantified ischemic stroke study in their picture analysis that the ischemic stroke keeps it producing. This will lead to the murder of blood bacteria on the cells of the brain. Imaging of magnetic resonance scans was widely used to identify brain magnetic strokes. An independent authority is in this study which may use the image processing techniques to diagnose stroke. There are six steps in this part. In the first step, MRI images retain knowledge. Pre-processing and filtrating should be carried out on raw information. In the third time period, the acquisition of a symmetrical image is traced by Midline. The image is bifurcated in the third step. In addition, neural networks are assigned to Phase 2 during the fifth phase of Imaging quality patterns in physical texture measurements, while normal and infected cerebral physiques have been set aside for the sixth. The downside is that in the early stages they can trace strokes. The approach of a project is simple and time consuming, as well as efficient [79].

4. Conclusions

In the chapter, a process was demonstrated for segmenting medical images of a stroke. Brain stroke segmentation, including pixels and morphology, consists of several segmentation steps and is a dynamic phase. The best way of exploring the MATLAB stroke with MRI images is to use clear images with more intellectual information provided by the MRI unit. Such approaches can discover different types of strokes at different levels of the brain. Researchers hope that, through this project, physicians will be able to understand MRI stroke photos.

Acknowledgements

This research was reinforced by the Applied Medical Science College of Majmaah University, Majmaah 11952, P.O box 1405, Saudi Arabia. We would like to express our gratitude toward RA (r.albaradie@mu.edu.sa) supervisor of the Stroke chair, Majmaah University and Dr. Khalid Bin Saad Al Murqrin, Rector, Majmaah University for providing the necessary support and assistance for completing this study This work was carried out under project number 38/130 Majmaah university.

Conflict of interest

The authors declare no conflict of interest.

Author details

Abdullah Alamoudi and Yousif Abdallah*
Department of Radiological Science and Medical Imaging, College of Applied Medical Science, Majmaah University, Saudi Arabia

*Address all correspondence to: y.yousif@mu.edu.sa

References

[1] G. Agam, D. Weiss, M. Soman, K. Arfanakis Probabilistic Brain Lesion Segmentation in DT-MRI (2007), pp. 89-92

[2] Ames III, R.L. Wright, M. Kowada, J.M. Thurston, G. Majno Cerebral ischemia. II. The no-reflow phenomenon The American Journal of Pathology, 52 (1968), pp. 437-453

[3] Anon.New resolution strategy for multi-scale reaction waves using time operator splitting and space adaptive multiresolution: application to human ischemic stroke, volume 34, EDP Sciences (2011)

[4] J.F. Arenillas, A. Rovira, C.A. Molina, E. Grivé, J. Montaner, J. Alvarez-SabínPrediction of early neurological deterioration using diffusion- and perfusion-weighted imaging in hyperacute middle cerebral artery ischemic stroke, Stroke, 33 (2002), pp. 2197-2203

[5] J. Astrup, L. Symon, N.M. Branston, N.A. LassenCortical evoked potential and extracellular K + and H + at critical levels of brain ischemia, Stroke, 8 (1977), pp. 51-57

[6] J. Astrup, B.K. Siesjö, L. SymonThresholds in cerebral ischemia — the ischemic penumbra

[7] Stroke, 12 (1981), pp. 723-725

[8] H. Bagher-Ebadian, K. Jafari-Khouzani, P.D. Mitsias, M. Lu, H. Soltanian-Zadeh, M. Chopp, J.R. EwingPredicting final extent of ischemic infarction using artificial neural network analysis of multi-parametric MRI in patients with stroke, PloS One, 6 (2011), p. e22626

[9] O.Y. Bang, J.L. Saver, B.H. Buck, J.R. Alger, S. Starkman, B. Ovbiagele, D. Kim, R. Jahan, G.R. Duckwiler, S.R. Yoon, F. Viñuela, D.S. Liebeskind, UCLA Collateral InvestigatorsImpact of collateral flow on tissue fate in acute ischaemic stroke. Journal of Neurology, Neurosurgery, and Psychiatry, 79 (2008), pp. 625-629

[10] P.A. Barber, D.G. Darby, P.M. Desmond, Q. Yang, R.P. Gerraty, D. Jolley, G.A. Donnan, B.M. Tress, S.M. DavisPrediction of stroke outcome with echoplanar perfusion- and diffusion-weighted MRI

[11] Neurology, 51 (1998), pp. 418-426

[12] R. Bonita Epidemiology of stroke Lancet, 339 (1992), pp. 342-344

[13] J. Braun, J. Bernarding, H.-C. Koennecke, K.-J. Wolf, T. TolxdorffFeature-based, automated segmentation of cerebral infarct patterns using T2- and diffusion-weighted imaging. Computer Methods in Biomechanics and Biomedical Engineering, 5 (2002), pp. 411-420

[14] T. Brott, J.R. Marler, C.P. Olinger, H.P. Adams Jr., T. Tomsick, W.G. Barsan, J. Biller, R. Eberle, V. Hertzberg, M. WalkerMeasurements of acute cerebral infarction: lesion size by computed tomography. Stroke, 20 (1989), pp. 871-875

[15] J.H. Burdette, A.D. Elster, P.E. RicciAcute cerebral infarction: quantification of spin-density and T2 shine-through phenomena on diffusion-weighted MR images. Radiology, 212 (1999), pp. 333-339

[16] R.A. Carano, K. Takano, K.G. Helmer, T. Tatlisumak, K. Irie, J.D. Petruccelli, M. Fisher, C.H. SotakDetermination of focal ischemic lesion volume in the rat brain using multispectral analysis. Journal of Magnetic Resonance Imaging, 8 (1998), pp. 1266-1278

[17] G. Chapuisat, M.A. Dronne, E. Grenier, M. Hommel, H. Gilquin, J.P. BoisselA global phenomenological model of ischemic stroke with stress on spreading depressions. Progress in Biophysics and Molecular Biology, 97 (2008), pp. 4-27

[18] G. Chapuisat, M.-A. Dronne, E. Grenier, M. Hommel, J.-P. BoisselIn silico study of the influence of intensity and duration of blood flow reduction on cell death through necrosis or apoptosis during acute ischemic stroke. Acta Biotheoretica, 58 (2010), pp. 171-190

[19] M. Chawla, S. Sharma, J. Sivaswamy, L. KishoreA method for automatic detection and classification of stroke from brain CT images Engineering in Medicine and Biology Society, 2009. EMBC 2009. Annual International Conference of the IEEE. IEEE (2009), pp. 3581-3584

[20] T. Chemmanam, B.C.V. Campbell, S. Christensen, Y. Nagakane, P.M. Desmond, C.F. Bladin, M.W. Parsons, C.R. Levi, P.A. Barber, G.A. Donnan, S.M. Davis, EPITHET InvestigatorsIschemic diffusion lesion reversal is uncommon and rarely alters perfusion–diffusion mismatch. Neurology, 75 (2010), pp. 1040-1047

[21] P. Choi, V. Srikanth, T. Phan"Fogging" resulting in normal MRI 3 weeks after ischaemic stroke. BMJ Case Reports, 2011 (2011)

[22] L. Contin, C. Beer, M. Bynevelt, H. Wittsack, G. GarridoSemi-automatic segmentation of core and penumbra regions in acute ischemic stroke: preliminary results. IWSSIP International Conference (2010)

[23] S.B. Coutts, J.E. Simon, A.I. Tomanek, P.A. Barber, J. Chan, M.E. Hudon, J.R. Mitchell, R. Frayne, M. Eliasziw, A.M. Buchan, A.M. DemchukReliability of assessing percentage of diffusion–perfusion mismatch. Stroke, 34 (2003), pp. 1681-1683

[24] K.A. Dani, R.G.R. Thomas, F.M. Chappell, K. Shuler, K.W. Muir, J.M. WardlawSystematic review of perfusion imaging with computed tomography and magnetic resonance in acute ischemic stroke: heterogeneity of acquisition and postprocessing parameters: a translational medicine research collaboration multicentre acute stroke imaging study. Stroke, 43 (2012), pp. 563-566

[25] P. Dastidar, T. Heinonen, J.P. Ahonen, M. Jehkonen, G. MolnárVolumetric measurements of right cerebral hemisphere infarction: use of a semiautomatic MRI segmentation technique. Computers in Biology and Medicine, 30 (2000), pp. 41-54

[26] B. Dawant, A. ZijdenbosImage segmentation. Handbook of Medical Imaging, 2 (2000), pp. 71-127

[27] M.-A. Dronne, J.-P. Boissel, E. Grenier, H. Gilquin, M. Cucherat, M. Hommel, E. Barbier, G. BriccaMathematical modelling of an ischemic stroke: an integrative approach. Acta Biotheoretica, 52 (2004), pp. 255-272

[28] M.-A. Dronne, J.-P. Boissel, E. GrenierA mathematical model of ion movements in grey matter during a stroke

[29] Journal of Theoretical Biology, 240 (2006), pp. 599-615

[30] T. Dumont, M. Duarte, S. Descombes, M. Dronne, M. Massot, V. LouvetSimulation of human ischemic stroke in realistic 3D geometry: a numerical strategy. Submitted to Bulletin of Math, Biology (2010)

[31] J. Duncan, N. AyacheMedical image analysis: progress over two decades

and the challenges ahead, pattern analysis and machine intelligence, IEEE Transactions on, 22 (2000), pp. 85-106

[32] V. Duval, S. Chabaud, P. Girard, M. Cucherat, M. Hommel, J.P. BoisselPhysiologically based model of acute ischemic stroke Journal of Cerebral Blood Flow and Metabolism, 22 (2002), pp. 1010-1018

[33] M.G. Dwyer, N. Bergsland, E. Saluste, J. Sharma, Z. Jaisani, J. Durfee, N. Abdelrahman, A. Minagar, R. Hoque, F.E. Munschauer III, R. ZivadinovApplication of hidden Markov random field approach for quantification of perfusion/diffusion mismatch in acute ischemic stroke. Neurological Research, 30 (2008), pp. 827-834

[34] G. Erus, E. Zacharaki, N. Bryan, C. DavatzikosLearning high-dimensional image statistics for abnormality detection on medical images. Computer Vision and Pattern Recognition Workshops (CVPRW), 2010 IEEE Computer Society Conference on. IEEE (2010), pp. 139-145

[35] Ford, H. An, K.V. LinDefining the ischemic penumbra using hyperacute neuroimaging: deriving quantitative ischemic thresholds. Translational Stroke Research (2012), pp. 1-7

[36] N. Ghosh, R. Recker, A. Shah, B. Bhanu, S.A. ObenausAutomated ischemic lesion detection in a neonatal model of hypoxic ischemic injury. Journal of Magnetic Resonance Imaging, 33 (2011), pp. 772-781

[37] N. Ghosh, Y. Sun, C.T. BhanuComputational analysis: a bridge to translational stroke treatment. Translational Stroke Research (2012), pp. 881-909

[38] V. Gupta, B. Prakash, W.L. NowinskiAutomatic and rapid identification of infarct slices and hemisphere in DWI scans. Academic Radiology, 15 (2008), pp. 24-39

[39] N. Hevia-Montiel, J.R. Jiménez-Alaniz, V. Medina-Bañuelos, O. Yáñez-Suárez, C. Rosso, Y. Samson, S. Baillet Robust nonparametric segmentation of infarct lesion from diffusion-weighted MR images. Conference Proceedings IEEE Engineering in Medicine and Biology Society, 2007 (2007), pp. 2102-2105

[40] E. Grenier, D. Bresch, M. Dronne, M. Hommel, J. BoisselA phenomenological model of the growth of the necrotic area in ischemic stroke. Mathematical and Computer Modelling, 51 (2010), pp. 1011-1025

[41] T. Heinonen, P. Dastidar, P. Kauppinen, J. Malmivuo, H. EskolaSemi-automatic tool for segmentation and volumetric analysis of medical images. Medical & Biological Engineering & Computing, 36 (1998), pp. 291-296

[42] N. Hevia-Montiel, C. Rosso, N. Chupin, S. Deltour, E. Bardinet, D. Dormont, Y. Samson, S. BailletAutomatic prediction of infarct growth in acute ischemic stroke from MR apparent diffusion coefficient maps. Academic Radiology, 15 (2008), pp. 77-83

[43] S. Huang, Q. Shen, T.Q. DuongArtificial neural network prediction of ischemic tissue fate in acute stroke imaging. Journal of Cerebral Blood Flow and Metabolism, 30 (2010), pp. 1661-1670

[44] M.A. Jacobs, R.A. Knight, H. Soltanian-Zadeh, Z.G. Zheng, A.V. Goussev, D.J. Peck, J.P. Windham, M. ChoppUnsupervised segmentation of multiparameter MRI in experimental cerebral ischemia with comparison to T2, diffusion, and ADC MRI parameters and histopathological validation. Journal of Magnetic Resonance Imaging, 11 (2000), pp. 425-437

[45] M.A. Jacobs, Z.G. Zhang, R.A. Knight, H. Soltanian-Zadeh, A.V. Goussev, D.J. Peck, M. ChoppA model for multiparametric MRI tissue characterization in experimental cerebral ischemia with histological validation in rat: part 1. Stroke, 32 (2001), pp. 943-949

[46] M.A. Jacobs, P. Mitsias, H. Soltanian-Zadeh, S. Santhakumar, A. Ghanei, R. Hammond, D.J. Peck, M. Chopp, S. PatelMultiparametric MRI tissue characterization in clinical stroke with correlation to clinical outcome: part 2. Stroke, 32 (2001), pp. 950-957

[47] J.R. James, K.K. Yoder, O. Osuntokun, A. Kalnin, A. Bruno, E.D. MorrisA supervised method for calculating perfusion/diffusion mismatch volume in acute ischemic stroke. Computers in Biology and Medicine, 36 (2006), pp. 1268-1287

[48] R. Józwiak, A.P. OstrekConceptual improvements in computer-aided diagnosis of acute stroke. Journal of Medical Informatics & Technologies Selected full texts, 17 (2011), pp. 191-199

[49] Y. Kabir, M. Dojat, B. Scherrer, F. Forbes, C. GarbayMultimodal MRI segmentation of ischemic stroke lesions Conference Proceedings IEEE Engineering in Medicine and Biology Society, 2007 (2007), pp. 1595-1598

[50] M.A. Kalafut, D.L. Schriger, J.L. Saver, S. StarkmanDetection of early CT signs of > 1/3 middle cerebral artery infarctions: interrater reliability and sensitivity of CT interpretation by physicians involved in acute stroke care. Stroke, 31 (2000), pp. 1667-1671

[51] Kane, T. Carpenter, F. Chappell, C. Rivers, P. Armitage, P. Sandercock, J. WardlawComparison of 10 different magnetic resonance perfusion imaging processing methods in acute ischemic stroke: effect on lesion size, proportion of patients with diffusion/perfusion mismatch, clinical scores, and radiologic outcomes. Stroke, 38 (2007), pp. 3158-3164

[52] D. Le Bihan, E. Breton, D. Lallemand, P. Grenier, E. Cabanis, M. Laval-JeantetMR imaging of intravoxel incoherent motions: application to diffusion and perfusion in neurologic disorders

[53] Radiology, 161 (1986), pp. 401-407

[54] C.B. Grandin, T.P. Duprez, A.M. Smith, C. Oppenheim, A. Peeters, A.R. Robert, G. CosnardWhich MR-derived perfusion parameters are the best predictors of infarct growth in hyperacute stroke? comparative study between relative and quantitative measurements. Radiology, 223 (2002), pp. 361-370

[55] T. Lelekov-Boissard, G. Chapuisat, J.-P. Boissel, E. Grenier, M.-A. DronneExploration of beneficial and deleterious effects of inflammation in stroke: dynamics of inflammation cells. Philosophical Transactions. Series A, Mathematical, Physical, and Engineering Sciences, 367 (2009), pp. 4699-4716

[56] W. Li, J. Tian, E. Li, J. DaiRobust unsupervised segmentation of infarct lesion from diffusion tensor MR images using multiscale statistical classification and partial volume voxel reclassification. NeuroImage, 23 (2004), pp. 1507-1518

[57] M. Li, L. Ai, H. He, Z. Zheng, B. Lv, W. Li, J. YiSegmentation of infarct in acute ischemic stroke from MR apparent diffusion coefficient and trace-weighted images. Proceedings of SPIE (2009)

[58] H.K. Ma, J.A. Zavala, L. Churilov, J. Ly, P.M. Wright, T.G. Phan, S. Arakawa, S.M. Davis, G.A. DonnanThe hidden mismatch: an explanation for infarct growth without perfusion-weighted

imaging/diffusion-weighted imaging mismatch in patients with acute ischemic stroke. Stroke, 42 (2011), pp. 662-668

[59] G. Majno, A. Ames, J. Chiang, R. WrightNo reflow after cerebral ischemia. Lancet, 290 (1967), pp. 569-570

[60] J.A. Maldjian, J. Chalela, S.E. Kasner, D. Liebeskind, J.A. DetreAutomated CT segmentation and analysis for acute middle cerebral artery stroke. AJNR. American Journal of Neuroradiology, 22 (2001), pp. 1050-1055

[61] Martel, S. Allder, G. Delay, P. Morgan, A. Moody Measurement of infarct volume in stroke patients using adaptive segmentation of diffusion weighted MR images. Medical Image Computing and Computer-Assisted Intervention–MICCAI'99. Springer (1999), pp. 22-31

[62] M. Matesin, S. Loncaric, D. PetravicA rule-based approach to stroke lesion analysis from CT brain images. Image and Signal Processing and Analysis, 2001. ISPA 2001. Proceedings of the 2nd International Symposium on. IEEE (2001), pp. 219-223

[63] M. Meilunas, A. Usinskas, R. Kirvaitis, R. DobrovolskisAutomatic contouring of segmented human brain ischemic stroke region on CT images. Mathematical Modelling and Analysis, 8 (2003), pp. 43-50

[64] M. Moseley, J. Kucharczyk, J. Mintorovitch, Y. Cohen, J. Kurhanewicz, N. Derugin, H. Asgari, D. NormanDiffusion-weighted MR imaging of acute stroke: correlation with T2-weighted and magnetic susceptibility-enhanced MR imaging in cats. American Journal of Neuroradiology, 11 (1990), pp. 423-429

[65] K.W. Muir, J. Baird-Gunning, L. Walker, T. Baird, M. McCormick, S.B. CouttsCan the ischemic penumbra be identified on noncontrast CT of acute stroke? Stroke, 38 (2007), pp. 2485-2490

[66] J. Murray. Mathematical Biology, Volume 2, Springer (2002)

[67] D.G. Na, V.N. Thijs, G.W. Albers, M.E. Moseley, M.P. MarksDiffusion-weighted MR imaging in acute ischemia: value of apparent diffusion coefficient and signal intensity thresholds in predicting tissue at risk and final infarct size. AJNR. American Journal of Neuroradiology, 25 (2004), pp. 1331-1336

[68] Y. Nagakane, S. Christensen, C. Brekenfeld, H. Ma, L. Churilov, M.W. Parsons, C.R. Levi, K.S. Butcher, A. Peeters, P.A. Barber, C.F. Bladin, D.A. De Silva, J. Fink, T.E. Kimber, D.W. Schultz, K.W. Muir, B.M. Tress, P.M. Desmond, S.M. Davis, G.A. Donnan, EPITHET InvestigatorsEPITHET: positive result after reanalysis using baseline diffusion-weighted imaging/perfusion-weighted imaging co-registration. Stroke, 42 (2011), pp. 59-64

[69] V. Nguyen, H. Pien, N. Menenzes, C. Lopez, C. Melinosky, O. Wu, A. Sorensen, G. Cooperman, H. Ay, W. KoroshetzStroke tissue outcome prediction using a spatially-correlated model. Program and Proceedings of PPIC, 8 (2008), pp. 238-241

[70] P. O'Brien, R.J. Sellar, J.M. WardlawFogging on T2-weighted MR after acute ischaemic stroke: how often might this occur and what are the implications? Neuroradiology, 46 (2004), pp. 635-641

[71] M.V.S.M.L.R.M. Olivot, J.M. Mlynash, G. AlbersOptimal Tmax threshold for predicting penumbral tissue in acute stroke Stroke, 40 (2009), pp. 469-475

[72] C. Oppenheim, Y. Grandin, C. Samson, A. Smith, T. Duprez, C. Marsault, G. CosnardIs there an apparent diffusion coefficient threshold in predicting tissue viability in hyperacute stroke? Stroke, 32 (2001), pp. 2486-2491

[73] J.R. Petrella, J.M. ProvenzaleMR perfusion imaging of the brain: techniques and applications. AJR. American Journal of Roentgenology, 175 (2000), pp. 207-219

[74] D. Pham, C. Xu, J. PrinceCurrent methods in medical image segmentation 1. Annual Review of Biomedical Engineering, 2 (2000), pp. 315-337

[75] T. Phan, G. Donnan, V. Srikanth, J. Chen, D. ReutensHeterogeneity in infarct patterns and clinical outcomes following internal carotid artery occlusion. Archives of Neurology, 66 (2009), p. 1523

[76] K.N. Bhanu Prakash, V. Gupta, M. Bilello, N.J. Beauchamp, W.L. NowinskiIdentification, segmentation, and image property study of acute infarcts in diffusion-weighted images by using a probabilistic neural network and adaptive Gaussian mixture model. Academic Radiology, 13 (2006), pp. 1474-1484

[77] J.-H. Rha, J.L. SaverThe impact of recanalization on ischemic stroke outcome: a meta-analysis. Stroke, 38 (2007), pp. 967-973

[78] C.S. Rivers, J.M. Wardlaw, P.A. Armitage, M.E. Bastin, T.K. Carpenter, V. Cvoro, P.J. Hand, M.S. DennisDo acute diffusion- and perfusion-weighted MRI lesions identify final infarct volume in ischemic stroke? Stroke, 37 (2006), pp. 98-104

[79] C.S. Rivers, J.M. Wardlaw, P.A. Armitage, M.E. Bastin, P.J. Hand, M.S. DennisAcute ischemic stroke lesion measurement on diffusion-weighted imaging—important considerations in designing acute stroke trials with magnetic resonance imaging. Journal of Stroke and Cerebrovascular Diseases, 16 (2007), pp. 64-70